TAKE CARE: THE HOME ENVIRONMENT GUIDE

One of seven empowering guides for true health and lasting joy

BY SARAH MORAN

Copyright © 2014 Sarah Moran
All rights reserved. No part may be reproduced in any form without permission from Take Care LLC. Reviewers may quote brief passages.

Designer: Micah Moran
Typeset in Bryant and Adelle

ISBN 978-1497575813

Take Care LLC
www.takecareguide.com

TABLE OF CONTENTS

7	About Take Care
10	Note to readers
15	**Home environment**
17	Jennifer's home environment story
19	Home environment introduction
29	**Home environment tips**
37	Air quality
40	Kitchen
43	Furniture
46	Electronics
47	Mattresses and bedding
50	Linens and bathroom
52	Paint
54	Floor and rugs
57	Cleaning products
61	Laundry
64	Air fresheners and candles
67	Toys and products for babies and children
72	Clothes
74	Pests
76	Lawn and garden
80	Garage
82	Cars
84	Countertops
85	Construction, home building and remodeling
88	Electromagnetic fields (EMF)

95	Resources
99	References
109	Experts' biographies
117	Acknowledgements
119	About the author

DEDICATION

For you, dear reader, for taking the time and energy to care for yourself. I believe everything that makes you healthier and happier serves everyone in your life and even the world at large.

ABOUT TAKE CARE

The Take Care series is a set of seven books covering multiple aspects of wellness: food, movement, body care products, home environment, sleep, balance and spirit. Each book has two parts. First, there's easy-to-read background with expert insights on the latest relevant research. Second, there are many practical tips, steps and ideas that make it easy for you to take action. Take Care is built on the following beliefs:

1. **Complete health has many components:** food, movement, body care products, home environment, sleep, balance and spirit. Together, they support all levels of well-being: body, mind, spirit.

2. **The aspects of good health connect and overlap.** That means every helpful step we take in one area of health creates a positive feedback loop and propels us toward further growth. The healthier we are, the healthier we keep getting. And it gets easier and faster as we progress.

    For example, people who write down what they're thankful for on a daily basis become more likely to exercise. People who exercise regularly sleep better. People who sleep better have more energy to exercise and make better choices about food. Healthy food, sleep and exercise all improve mood. A positive mood energizes people to create more of what they want in life. And so on.

3. **The roots of true health and lasting joy are simple, unchanging and intuitive.** The same basic principles of good health apply to all the different types of health. For instance, staying closer to nature is better. Man-made chemicals—whether they're in our food, mattresses or soap—often cause trouble for our health.

Additionally, people thrive when they follow the rhythms of nature and alternate between cycles of activity and rest, growth and integration. This is true whether you're talking about intervals in an exercise program, carving out a dedicated time to sleep at night or managing your daily schedule so you have downtime to reflect and recharge.

4. **The same healthy choices help prevent or improve numerous diseases and conditions.** And the same unhealthy choices increase our risk. Although genetics and other uncontrollable factors certainly play a role, there's still a lot we can do for our well-being.

    For example, eating well, getting adequate sleep and reducing chemical exposure all help maintain a healthy body weight. And protect against cancer. And boost fertility. And lower blood pressure. And improve mental health. And so on.

5. **Good health care is like good gardening—if you really want to eliminate a weed, you need to get at the roots. And if you want your flowers to blossom, you need to be aware of the environment in which you're planting them.** If we fail to address the root cause of a health issue and instead focus only on treating, masking or covering up its symptoms, the problem is bound to pop up again. It's like trying to get dandelions out of your yard by chopping off the flowers on top—a short-term "solution" at best. And, just like a good gardener knows a plant needs the right soil, sun and water to thrive, our thoughtful choices regarding food, movement, body care products, home environment, sleep, balance and spirit help us to be at our best.

6. **True health benefits all the dimensions of being human—body, mind and spirit.** Healthy is happy. And happy is healthy. Health has nothing to do with counting calories and depriving yourself of tasty food. Nor is it about trudging along for a certain number of minutes on a treadmill. Rather, true health is about eating foods that energize you. It's about moving your body in a way that helps you feel good and allows you to keep doing the things you want to do. True health is rejuvenating, fulfilling and joyful.

I hope the Take Care books will inform, empower and inspire you to continually make your life healthier, happier and easier.

Wishing you the best,

Sarah

NOTE TO READERS

Keep this in mind as you read and learn:

1. **Be empowered, not overwhelmed. Inspired, not worried.** This information is here to serve you. A lot of things are outside our control, including experiences and choices from the past—so let them go. Focus on what is in your sphere of influence, given your current circumstances. Being well informed can give you momentum to take action as you're ready and able.

2. **Trust yourself. As you decide what healthy changes to make, take the step you feel like taking instead of the step you think you should take.** Deep down, you'll know where to begin and what will serve you best right now. If a particular topic piques your interest or a certain action seems energizing, go there and do that. If you follow your intuition, you're more likely to get on the right path sooner and to be motivated about progressing.

3. **Take small steps. Or, in some cases, go big! Just take your next right step.** Nobody's perfect, and you don't have to change everything at once. For many people, it's best to set reasonable goals and take things one step at a time. But you might be a person who does better making sweeping changes with deep focus. If your circumstances allow it, go for it. You know yourself best, so do what you sense to be the most effective strategy for you.

4. **Remember that the healthier you are, the easier it is to listen to your body.** When we're polluting or draining ourselves in any sense, our bodies can't communicate with us as well. But

every step you take toward better health further clears your whole being: body, mind, spirit and energy. With every degree of improvement, you become more in tune with yourself.

5. **As in all things, balance is essential.** Our focus naturally evolves throughout different periods and stages of life. What you're able to cultivate and what you need to compromise on are different as an adolescent, a student, a parent of a newborn and a grandparent. Consider what you're able to do for your health and happiness given your current circumstances and work on that.

6. **Use support as you wish.** Reach out to kindred spirits who can support your ongoing journey toward higher levels of well-being. Find experts and health practitioners who can help you continually go deeper. Tell supportive family and friends about your aspirations.

DISCLAIMER

This book contains my opinions and ideas. Although I work hard to be correct and current, I make no guarantees the information, opinions or statements are accurate or up to date. I'm continually learning, and health information constantly evolves. One expert's views might be different than another's. I welcome comments, suggestions and corrections.

My intent is to offer general information to help people who are interested in making healthier choices and living more consciously. This book is offered and sold with the understanding that I am not providing personal health advice. The reader should consult with a health professional before incorporating suggestions, whether direct or implied, from this content. The reader should not rely on this information as an alternative to seeking help from a medical professional, nor should the reader delay seeking medical attention as a result of information here.

The opinions in Take Care content are mine alone and do not represent the views of any of my past or current clients or employers. Under no circumstances shall I, Take Care LLC, or any contributors be responsible for damages resulting directly or indirectly from this content. This material shall not be used in any legal capacity whatsoever.

I endorse resources, brands and products only because they have met certain high standards. These mentions are based purely on merit and are intended to help the reader find solutions and make improvements more easily.

Thank you,
Sarah Moran
Take Care LLC

Topic IV

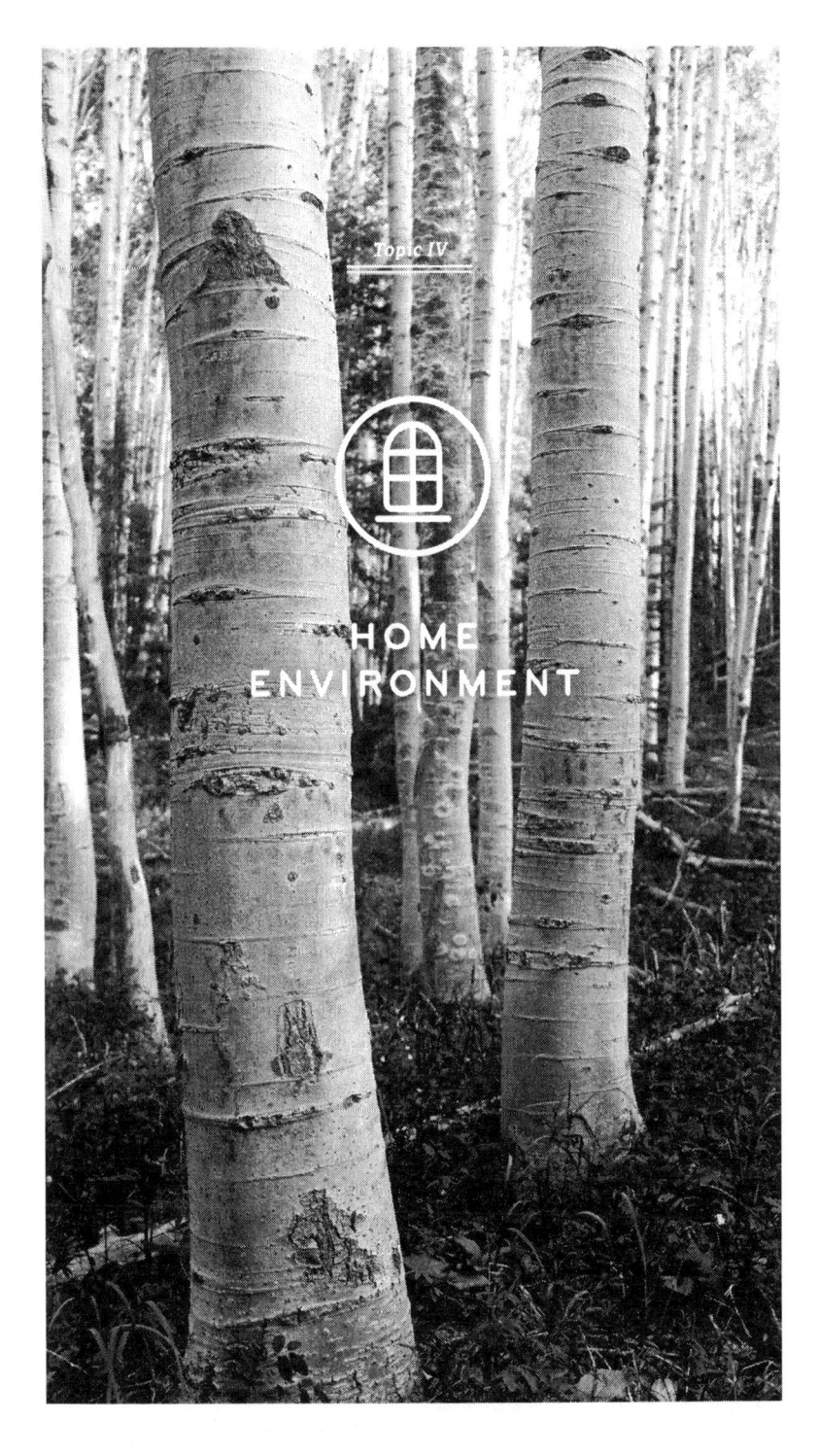

HOME ENVIRONMENT

JENNIFER'S HOME ENIVRONMENT STORY

From Jennifer, age 44

Like most people, we used to just buy the popular brands of things for our home. The easiest way to describe it is that we walked into a big box store and bought what was on the shelf.

Later, my husband and I were going through a long run of infertility and treatment for it, so I started looking around my environment and wondering about how I could affect my own fertility. Then when I was pregnant, I heard different things about chemicals in products and how they could affect the baby. I wasn't sure what to make of it all, and I didn't always believe it. But I started paying more attention.

The biggest trigger of all was once we had our baby. I'm embarrassed to say it now, but I was using a popular brand of deodorizer that I'd spray around my son's diaper pail because I thought it would kill germs and keep the smell away. When my son was 2, he got a cold that wouldn't go away, and he had a cough for something like six months. The doctor called it "suspected asthma." My son was put on an intensive medication and had to use a nebulizer. At the time, we didn't really know how to question that or what to do about it.

That's when I really started learning about chemicals and how they affect health. The mainstream media only touches on this a little bit, but when you look closer, the research and studies are pretty astonishing. I realized that these chemicals coming into our bodies could have so many more consequences than what we know at this point.

I essentially said, "That's it, I'm peeling away anything that's controversial and cleaning everything out in the house." It didn't happen all at once, of course, and with some items, it takes a monetary commitment too.

First, I stopped using the deodorizer in my son's room and started making all my own cleaning products. We also stopped using anything with bleach or antibacterial soaps, neither of which is necessary. We got rid of everything plastic that we could, especially storage containers for food and the PVC plastic that's in some baby toys and shower curtains and raincoats. We switched to glass baby bottles and stainless-steel sippy cups. I also changed cookware and got rid of our nonstick stuff and went to cast iron—which we love cooking with!—and stainless-steel pans. We also eventually bought a new mattress for my son. Although it wasn't organic, it was a much cleaner version than what he had before. And now we don't buy anything with a scent unless the fragrance comes from an essential oil.

As soon as we got the gunk out of the house, especially the deodorizer, my son's cough went away. He no longer had "suspected asthma," and he didn't need the medication or nebulizer anymore. My allergies also got dramatically better.

When I used popular cleaning products, I'd get headaches or my eyes would water or my nose would run. That should be a red flag for all of us. With my homemade cleaning products, none of that happens.

After learning more about this and seeing the difference in my own family, I believe in this so much. If people can make small changes now, it will help in the short term and the long term. At the end of the day, you have to be your own advocate and stand up for integrity in the products you purchase. If you just buy cheap all the time, that's what you'll get. It shouldn't be about getting the best deal; it should be about finding products with integrity that work for your family.

This can feel overwhelming for people, but I'd say just start with one thing you know you can do and go from there. It doesn't all have to happen at once, but if you start with one thing, the next thing will come easier.

HOME ENVIRONMENT INTRODUCTION

· · · · · · ·

"The strength of a nation derives from the integrity of the home."
—CONFUCIUS

At its best, our home is a place we look forward to after a long day, a place we feel relaxed, comfortable and safe. When we think of home, certainly the last thing that should come to mind is "health hazard." But the simple choices we make about what everyday products we use—furniture, mattresses, cleaning products, paint, phones, electronics, candles and even toys—can determine whether our home is a breath of fresh air or a bastion of funk.

Consumers' choices about seemingly innocent products have led to indoor air being typically two to five times (and even up to 100 times) more polluted than outdoor air, according to the Environmental Protection Agency.[1] And mounting scientific evidence links everyday chemicals used in consumer products to a range of health conditions, including diabetes, high blood pressure and cancer.

WHAT HOMES CAN HARBOR

People absorb household chemicals in numerous ways: through the air they breathe, the way they prepare their food and even the products they touch.

One big health issue has to do with volatile organic compounds (VOCs), which are invisible particles that evaporate off products and into the air you breathe. All sorts of items and materials let off VOCs, sometimes for years or even decades: furniture, carpet, glues, cleaning supplies, shower curtains and paint. According to the EPA, concentrations of VOCs indoors are consistently higher than outdoors—up to 10 times so. VOCs lead to short- and long-term health problems, everything from headaches and fatigue to cancer and damage to the liver, kidneys and central nervous system.[2]

Another major problem comes in the form of dust. In addition to shed skin cells and microscopic mites, dust often consists of tiny particles that migrate off all kinds of products, including furniture, plastic toys, carpet and paint. Many harmful chemicals aren't bound, which means they easily travel off and through products. The end result? Household dust that contains carcinogens, flame retardants, hormone-disrupting chemicals and heavy metals, such as lead. Dust settles in thin layers all around the house: in heating and ventilation systems, on the floors and atop furniture. People, especially babies and children, ingest dust mainly through hand-to-mouth contact and inhalation.

Flame-retardant chemicals are one of the big health concerns, and they're added to many household items: crib mattresses, furniture, electronics, fabrics, blankets, drapes, kids' pajamas, hair dryers, electronics and more.

One study, funded by the National Institute of Environmental Health Sciences, showed that toddlers have significant exposure to flame retardants through dust.[3]

According to a recent report from the Green Science Policy Institute, "Toddlers have three to four times the levels of toxic flame retardants in their bodies compared to their parents. These chemicals pose a serious hazard to pregnant women and young children who are the most vulnerable to endocrine disruptors, carcinogens, mutagens, and neurological and reproductive toxins."[4]

Flame retardants are in pretty much everyone's body, according to Centers for Disease Control and Prevention (CDC) research. And contamination levels have risen sharply over the past couple of decades.[5] One study showed that levels of flame retardants in breast milk had risen 60-fold from 1972 to 1997.[6] Research shows flame retardants can disrupt the hormone system, decrease fertility[7] and lower thyroid hormone levels in pregnant women.[8] Exposure in utero is associated with poorer attention, fine-motor skills and cognition in grade-school children.[9]

GLOSSARY

Volatile organic compounds (VOCs) *are invisible gases made up of a variety of chemicals. VOCs occur when products—solid or liquid—release tiny particles into the air. They lead to short- and long-term health consequences.*

Off-gassing *is the process of VOCs releasing or evaporating into the air. Some products off-gas for years.*

Carcinogens *are substances known to play a role in causing cancer.*

Flame retardants *are substances—usually chemical in nature—that delay by a few seconds how long it takes for a material to ignite.*

Endocrine-disruptors, or hormone-disrupting chemicals, *mimic human hormones and throw off your body's natural hormone system, also known as the endocrine system.*

Genes *are pieces of DNA that carry specific instructions to cells. Genes are the blueprints that help determine just about everything for people: looks, skills, behavior, responses, how their body functions and how likely they are to develop certain diseases and conditions.*

Gene expression *refers to how your cells only express, or "turn on," a portion of their genes at different times. Other genes remain unexpressed, or "turned off." Hormonal changes, environmental triggers and lifestyle choices can determine whether a gene is turned on or off, as well as how the gene functions. These changes can then trigger or prevent diseases and conditions.*

Synthetic products *are man-made materials or ingredients. They're often created by using a chemical process.*

CONTAMINANTS LINKED TO MANY MODERN DISEASES

A home certainly doesn't have to be so polluted—informed consumers can make better choices for healthier homes, says David O. Carpenter, M.D., director for the Institute for Health and the Environment at the University of Albany in New York.

"Fifty years ago or so, we used natural materials like cotton, linen, wool and real wood, but today, almost everything is made from oil-based products: plastics, artificial fabrics and synthetic materials," he says. "Now there are 85,000 man-made chemicals in our environment, and it's becoming apparent that exposure to them is increasing our risk for disease.

"We're finding that environmental exposure to chemicals has a strong influence on the rates of common diseases that people have never considered to be related, like high blood pressure, diabetes and thyroid disease. Many chemicals also make it harder to learn and trigger abnormal attention spans or behavior problems, which is especially concerning for children," Carpenter says. "The effect that common chemicals have on health is incredibly important, but people are generally just not aware."

The President's Cancer Panel, after two years of research, reported in 2010 that "the true burden of environmentally induced cancer has been grossly underestimated" and that "the public remains unaware of many common environmental carcinogens." The panel added, "The American people—even before they are born—are bombarded continually with myriad combinations of these dangerous exposures."[10]

Research shows chemical exposure is contributing to other modern diseases and health conditions. Consider the following:

- There's a "striking" relationship between the concentration of certain pollutants in a person's body and the prevalence of diabetes, according to a study from the National Health and Nutrition Examination Survey.[11]
- Lead exposures, "even at levels well below the current U.S. occupational exposure limit guidelines," are associated with higher blood pressure and risk for hypertension, according to a study in The Journal of the American Medical Association.[12] Another study links arsenic exposure to hypertension,[13] and another shows PCB exposure is strongly associated with higher systolic and diastolic blood pressure.[14]

- Research shows an association between children's exposure to phthalates—a class of man-made chemicals widely used in products such as synthetic flooring, shower curtains, wall coverings and shampoo—and increased body mass index (BMI) and waist circumference.[15]
- The White House Task Force on Childhood Obesity report says that exposure to certain chemicals may play a role in childhood obesity: "Such chemicals may promote obesity by increasing the number of fat cells, changing the amount of calories burned at rest, altering energy balance, and altering the body's mechanisms for appetite and satiety."[16]
- A study supported by the National Institute of Environmental Health Sciences shows a link between exposure to polyfluoroalkyl chemicals (PFCs)—found in stain-resistant coating, food packaging and nonstick kitchen products—and attention deficit hyperactivity disorder (ADHD) in children.[17]

CHEMICALS CAN CHANGE YOUR GENES

How is it that chemicals can trigger disease? Carpenter explains that chemicals can change how a person's genes are expressed. For instance, a chemical exposure could affect the gene that controls a person's metabolism and cause his or her metabolism to slow. Or if someone has the genetic potential for a certain disease, chemical exposure could cause that gene to "turn on," thereby activating a disease that might have otherwise never actually developed for that individual. "Modern genetic techniques are showing that hundreds of genes can be changed as a result of chemical exposures," Carpenter says.

The fact that chemicals can change gene expression—leading to the eventual development of disease and adverse health conditions—is concerning enough. It's even more daunting when you consider that a person's exposure can change the genetic code for his or her children, grandchildren and great-grandchildren.[18]

EXPOSURE BEGINS BEFORE BIRTH

It's well established that babies—even before they're born—are contaminated with chemicals, and it's affecting their health.

- One study by the Environmental Working Group and Rachel's Network found up to 232 toxic chemicals in the umbilical cord blood of a sample of newborn babies. Among the chemicals were those used in metal food cans and plastic bottles; flame retardants; chemicals used to make nonstick, grease-, stain- and water-resistant coatings; synthetic fragrances and polychlorinated biphenyls (PCBs), which are now banned from being manufactured in the U.S. but have been used for years in lubricants, insulating materials and caulk.[19]
- Another study showed that baby boys who were exposed to phthalates while still in the womb showed various signs of delayed sexual development, including incomplete testicular development and smaller penis volume.[20]
- One analysis of multiple studies on parental pesticide exposure and childhood cancer concluded that "the incidence of childhood cancer does appear to be associated with parental exposure during the prenatal period."[21]

Studies confirm that most of us are taking in chemicals that are found in everyday household products. Research by the CDC shows that:[22]
- More than 90 percent of people sampled were contaminated with BPA, which is commonly used in metal-can lining and hard-plastic water bottles.
- Pretty much everyone has some flame-retardant chemicals in their bodies.
- Most people show exposure to perfluorooctanoic acid, which indicates they're taking in the chemicals used to make nonstick coatings.

SMALL DOSES STILL MATTER, AND THEY'RE ADDING UP

It would be easy to dismiss the data on widespread contamination by surmising that many of these chemicals are present only in small doses. How much does the off-gassing from a plastic shower curtain really matter? Or the flame retardants on your sofa? Or the chemicals that slough off from the plastic toys kids play with?

Research shows that low-dose exposures are a serious concern, and experts are warning about the harmful cumulative and synergistic effects.

It's not surprising that the mixture of everyday chemicals could make for an even more toxic cocktail. Consider one study of 10 pesticides and their impact in an aquatic environment. The study exposed various species of aquatic life, including zooplankton, gray tree frogs and leopard frogs, to low doses of 10 pesticides one at a time. Administered individually, each pesticide wiped out varying percentages of different species. But when all 10 pesticides were mixed together and administered, they killed 99 percent of one species.[23]

One large class of commonly used chemicals is known as endocrine-disrupting chemicals because they disrupt the body's endocrine, or hormone, system. The hormone system is responsible for many lifelong vital functions, including growth, cell division, stress response, metabolism, blood sugar, behavior and intelligence, as well as the development of the brain, reproductive system and nervous system.

A group of experts on endocrine disruption recently reviewed the studies and data on the effects of endocrine-disrupting chemicals, referred to here as "EDCs." They concluded that "there is now substantial evidence that low doses of EDCs have adverse effects on human health" and that "these recent studies have suggested wide-ranging effects of EDCs on the general population."[24]

The scientists also said that "dozens if not hundreds of environmental chemicals are regularly detected in human tissues and fluids, yet very little is known about how these chemicals act in combination. Several studies indicate that EDCs can have additive or even synergistic effects, and thus these mixtures are likely to have unexpected and unpredictable effects on animals and humans."

Theo Colborn, founder of The Endocrine Disruption Exchange, based in Paonia, Colo., was one of the scientists on the review. "We know that even in minute amounts, such as parts per billion or parts per trillion, these chemicals can interfere with every major organ system," she says. Besides, Colborn adds, even if a small amount were to be proven safe, people are surrounded by multiple products every day.

Linda Birnbaum, Ph.D., director of the National Institute of Environmental Health Sciences of the National Institutes of Health, wrote in a 2012 editorial that "the mere presence of a chemical in humans is not necessarily cause for concern. What is concerning is the increasing number of epidemiological studies showing associations between the concentration of these chemicals in the general population and adverse health end points."[25]

OBSTACLES TO SAFER PRODUCTS

With alarm bells ringing and researchers and other health professionals voicing concern, why hasn't more been done to protect consumers from chemicals in household products?

Part of the problem is that there's a massive number of man-made chemicals that have come into our lives in the last several decades, says Richard J. Jackson, M.D., M.P.H., a pediatrician and professor and chair of Environmental Health Sciences at UCLA's Fielding School of Public Health.

"There are 85,000-some chemicals being used out there, and in the U.S. they're treated as innocent until proven guilty," he says. "Proving them guilty and worthy of removal is extremely difficult." Europeans, he points out, have moved to requiring a new chemical be proven safe before it can be put to market.

"Another problem is that damage from early exposures are often unclear—a young body is better able to mask or overcome exposure," he says. "It's not until later in life that vulnerabilities and the consequences of that exposure start to emerge."

The time it takes for diseases and conditions to develop (often decades) adds another challenge to attempts to prove a chemical is not safe, says Carpenter. Plus, he adds, there are numerous conflicts of interest in this area: If a chemical is banned, industries have to spend a lot of time and money reformulating products; consumers today are used to cheap goods; and doctors and other health professionals are so busy trying to make people well that they often don't have time to look into what's causing disease and illness in the first place or to keep up with the latest research.

CHEMICALS' MUCH YOUNGER COUSIN: ELECTROMAGNETIC FIELDS (EMF)

Another area of growing concern is exposure to electromagnetic fields (EMFs). Newer technologies, such as cellphones and WiFi, carry powerful waves that emit EMFs and can penetrate the human brain, organs and other tissues.

EMFs have the potential to interfere with how cells in your body communicate with one another, inhibit your cells' ability to detoxify and repair themselves, create a stress response in the body and affect hormone levels.

Research in the area of EMF exposure and health is in its infancy, however, and its study is challenged by conflicts of interest, conflicting results and ever-changing, increasingly powerful technology.

Some of the health consequences, including cancer, can take decades to develop, for instance, so they may not be captured by studies that span shorter periods of time. Nonetheless, there are already plenty of studies that indicate EMF exposure puts people in danger, including those showing an increased risk for brain tumors[26][27][28][29], serious damage to human sperm,[30][31][32] and behavior problems in children.[33]

One respected review analyzed multiple long-term epidemiological studies and determined that using a cell phone for 10 years or more "approximately doubles the risk of being diagnosed with a brain tumor on the same ('ipsilateral') side of the head as that preferred for cell phone use."[34]

"EMF exposure and all the other aspects of a healthy home can really affect your vitality," says Kara Parker, M.D., who practices with the Hennepin County Medical Center in Minneapolis. "The home environment is a cornerstone—I often wish I could do home visits to see what's in a patient's environment that could be negatively affecting their health."

The problem of exposure to chemicals and EMFs can be overwhelming and complicated, but the good news is that your home is an area over which you have some real control. Because it's probably a place you spend a good portion of your time, the choices you make toward a healthier home can make an important difference.

Topic IV

TIPS & RESOURCES

HOME ENVIRONMENT TIPS

The pages that follow include about 200 practical tips, solutions and ideas for a healthier home and a healthier you. Think of this as a menu to pick and choose from. Begin with whatever sounds best to you. And then when you're ready, challenge yourself to try the next thing that sounds good.

1. **Watch out for VOCs.** These invisible particles off-gas from products like furniture, cleaning supplies, air fresheners, shower curtains and more. They're often found in products made of synthetic substances, such as plastic, foam and other man-made materials. If you can smell something (that new-car smell or your shower curtain), you're probably inhaling VOCs. But just because your nose adapts or the smell goes away doesn't mean the item has stopped off-gassing—some products release VOCs for years. VOCs can cause all kinds of health effects: eye, nose and throat irritation; headaches; fatigue; allergic reactions; nausea; dizziness; and even cancer.[35] Read on for specifics about finding products without VOCs.

2. **Look into whether (and which) flame retardants are used.** Flame retardant chemicals are widely used and are commonplace in upholstered furniture, kids' mattresses, carpet padding, draperies, high chairs, nursing pillows and more. If a product has a label that says it meets California Technical Bulletin 117 (TB117), then it probably contains potentially harmful flame retardant chemicals. Many products without the label also contain these chemicals.

   If an item is made with polyurethane foam, there's a good chance the piece has flame retardants (unless it was made prior to 1975, when TB117 was enacted and widely adopted). Remember that the older an item gets, the more it breaks down and easily lets these chemicals loose.

Some flame retardants have proven so hazardous that they've been banned from the marketplace. For example, one type known as PBDEs should not be found in foam products made in 2005 onward. But plenty of other dangerous flame retardants are still in use. Some use antimony, a chemical shown to cause skin and eye problems for humans when inhaled, as well as respiratory, cardiovascular and kidney problems in animal studies.[36]

Many experts believe that the risks posed by chemical flame retardants outweigh any potential benefit they might offer in briefly delaying a flame from igniting. Research supporting this point continues to mount, and recent reforms mean more flame-retardant-free items will likely become available.

Generally, you can also play it safer by avoiding polyurethane foam in products and opting for items made with natural materials such as wool, down or solid wood. Wool is naturally flame retardant. Hydrated silica is another safer, more natural choice for a flame retardant.

The Green Science Policy Institute has up-to-date information and tips about flame retardant chemicals: *www.greensciencepolicy.org*.

The Center for Environmental Health lists brands that make flame retardant-free furniture and products: *www.ceh.org/campaigns/flame-retardants/ceh-action/finding-safer-products/*.

3. **Dust isn't just a housekeeping issue—it often contains hazardous materials.** Research shows that dust often contains various unhealthy materials that have sloughed off household items. Lead, formaldehyde and flame retardants are frequently found in dust. Everyone inhales dust throughout the day, but babies take in much more dust than adults.[37] This is because babies and kids breathe in more air than adults per body weight, they regularly play on the floor where they're in contact with dust and they have more hand-to-mouth behaviors. Remember also that when you touch chemicals, some can be absorbed into your body through your skin, which is permeable. Dust regularly with a damp rag. Clean dust from floors using a vacuum with a HEPA filter and a damp mop.

4. **Avoid products that say they're nonstick, stain-repellant, grease-repellant, wrinkle-resistant or insect-repelling.** These products are likely coated in chemicals, including those in a class known as perfluorochemicals (PFCs). Some types of PFCs, including PFOA and PFOS, have proven so harmful that they're finally being phased out (although that doesn't protect you from products manufactured before the bans are effective or from other PFCs that might be just as dangerous but haven't been banned from the market). PFCs can stay in the human body for several years. Animal studies show that "some PFCs disrupt normal endocrine activity; reduce immune function; cause adverse effects on multiple organs, including the liver and pancreas; and cause developmental problems in rodent offspring exposed in the womb," according to the National Institute of Environmental Health Sciences.[38]

5. **Maintain a no-shoes-in-the-house policy (it's for your health, not your floors).** When people wear shoes in the house, they track in a lot of unsavory guests: chemicals, oils, pesticides, dog doo-doo, dander and so on. Removing shoes at the door keeps your house much healthier and cleaner. The Environmental Protection Agency (EPA) recommends removing shoes at the door.[39]

6. **Choose solid wood and avoid fiberboard, particleboard and pressed wood.** If it's not solid wood, an item is much more likely to emit VOCs from the chemical finishes, glues and adhesives used to make it. Imitation wood often contains formaldehyde, a probable human carcinogen,[40] and flame retardants, which may disrupt your hormone system,[41] decrease fertility,[42] impact thyroid hormones[43] and negatively affect intelligence and behavior.[44]

7. **Look for a safe and natural wood finish, that is, a water-based finish or one that uses certain plant oils.** This could include walnut, linseed and tung oil or beeswax. If a wood product is certified by FSC (Forest Stewardship Council), it uses safer finishes.

8. **Choose natural fibers, such as cotton, linen, wool, cashmere, bamboo or silk. Avoid plastic, vinyl and foam.** Natural materials

are all that was used for most of human history. They're safe, don't contaminate the air or environment and don't emit VOCs. (Some people are allergic to wool, however). Man-made products, such as plastic, vinyl and foam, can continuously shed and emit chemicals.

9. **Choose untreated, organic fibers and fabrics whenever possible (GOTS-certified products are a great choice).** This will reduce your exposure to chemicals that are used to grow conventional crops and to treat and finish fabric. Cotton is one of the dirtiest crops around—it's usually heavily doused in pesticides, and the pesticides it uses are particularly hazardous. According to the Natural Resources Defense Council, "about a third of a pound of chemical pesticides and fertilizers go into each pound of conventionally-grown American cotton."[45] In addition, a recent report by the Environmental Justice Foundation states that "cotton accounts for 16 percent of the global insecticide releases – more than any other single crop."[46]

   Buying an organic, untreated cotton mattress will cut your exposure to those pesticides and other chemical finishes that are commonly used on conventional cotton.

   Note that wool that isn't labeled organic might undergo chemical processes before being made into a mattress or bedding. Reduce your exposure by choosing organic.

   GOTS (Global Organic Textile Standard) certification is an international standard that tells you a product meets a variety of standards for health and the environment.

   Another good certification for fabrics and textiles is called OEKO-TEX. If you see this on a label, it means that the product has been tested—and does not contain—certain harmful substances.

10. **Look for products that use eco-friendly or "low-impact" dyes.** Instead of using synthetic chemicals, these dyes color products with extracts from natural materials, such as vegetables, plants or clay. If a product is GOTS-certified, that means it doesn't use certain harsh chemicals in dyes.

11. **Skip household products that say they're antibacterial.** They're often made using triclosan, which is known to alter

hormone regulation in animals.[47] Lab studies have linked triclosan to cancer, developmental defects, and liver and inhalation toxicity.[48] Other studies, including one from the American Medical Association, show that antibacterial soaps are no more effective at killing germs than regular soap and water, and these antibacterial agents are contributing to bacterial resistance.[49][50] A CDC study showed that 75 percent of Americans are contaminated with triclosan.[51]

12. **Choose products without phthalates.** This class of chemicals is commonly used in food packaging, toys, cleaning products, soaps, shower curtains, floors and wall coverings. Many phthalates are known to be hormone-disrupting chemicals. A CDC study testing for the presence of seven phthalates in Americans showed that 75 percent of the subjects had four of the phthalates in their bodies.[52] Phthalates are linked to delayed sexual development and smaller penis volume in baby boys exposed in utero;[53] asthma and allergies and problems with neurodevelopment, reproductive hormone levels and thyroid function;[54] increases in aggression, depression and attention problems;[55] DNA damage in men's sperm[56] and an increased body mass index (BMI) and waist circumference.[57]

13. **Care about cleanliness.** The cleaner you keep your home, the more you'll cut back on allergens and irritants.

14. **Learn to make your own cleaning products, laundry detergents and air fresheners.** This gives you full control over ingredients. Recipes are often easy to make and can save a lot of money. You can use hydrogen peroxide or vinegar as natural disinfectants, for instance. Read on for more details.

15. **Learn about electromagnetic fields (EMFs) and take steps to minimize your exposure.** See page 88 for dozens of tips.

16. **Hire a building biologist.** These professionals come to your home to evaluate and make suggestions to improve air quality, EMF exposure and other aspects of a healthy home environment.

17. **Look for products certified by Green Seal or GREENGUARD.** See www.greenseal.org and www.greenguard.org. Certified products have met standards for health, safety and the environment.

18. **Look for products labeled as "USDA certified biobased product."** This government certification means that the item is made from at least 25 percent biobased content. According to the program, "A biobased product is a product that is determined by the USDA to be a commercial or industrial product (other than food or feed) that is composed, in whole or in significant part, of biological products, including renewable domestic agricultural materials forestry materials, and marine and animal materials." See www.biopreferred.gov for more details.

19. **Take advantage of helpful resources,** including the Environmental Working Group's website, www.ewg.org, as well as the websites www.healthystuff.org and earth911.com for tips, reports, rankings, studies and background on various consumer products.

20. **Bookmark and frequent the website of author Debra Lynn Dadd,** at www.debralynndadd.com and her list of healthier consumer products at www.debralynndadd.com/debraslist. Her comprehensive guide "Debra's List" allows you to look up the best brands and websites in all sorts of categories, including air filters, art supplies, cleaning, interior decorating, textiles and more.

21. **Remember that if it's bad for the environment, it's probably bad for your health.** It makes sense that something that's harmful for the rest of creation (plants, animals, water, soil and air) is likely bad for people. In addition, the consequences of harm to the Earth, such as polluted water, soil and air, come back around and cause problems for human health. Spend a moment thinking about how a product was manufactured or how it works, and it should be relatively easy to sort out what items you'd want to bring into your home and which you'd rather not buy and support. Use your consumer dollars to vote for a healthier future.

AIR QUALITY

• • • • • • •

"For in the final analysis, our most basic common link is that we all inhabit this small planet. We all breathe the same air. We all cherish our children's futures. And we are all mortal."

— JOHN F. KENNEDY

The air quality in your home is based on many things, including the products and furnishings you choose, the materials that were used to build your place and how you keep your house clean. Although chemical exposure is one important piece of a healthy home, problems such as mold and dust mites also need to be looked at. Poor air quality from natural and man-made sources can lead to everything from asthma and allergies to cancer and organ damage.

1. **Avoid volatile organic compounds (VOCs).** Choose products without these unhealthy chemicals. That generally means limiting your use of synthetic materials and plastics and opting for natural materials, such as wood, stone, cotton and wool.

2. **Invest in your air, heat and ventilation system.** Make sure you have a good-quality, well-functioning, up-do-date central heating, ventilation and air quality (HVAC) system. One with a washable or replaceable HEPA (high-efficiency particulate air) filter is best for removing small particles, such as dust, dander and pollen. Use an activated carbon filter too in order to capture certain chemicals

and gasses, including VOCs, that are too small for even the HEPA filter to catch.

3. **Make sure your ventilation system is working well.** This will help keep moisture, along with mildew and mold, from becoming a problem. Good ventilation is especially important in moisture-prone areas, such as bathrooms, kitchens and laundry rooms.

4. **Keep an eye out for other places water can creep in.** Fix leaks and cracks as soon as you see them to keep mildew and mold at bay.

5. **Maintain proper humidity levels: usually 30 to 50 percent.** You can measure the humidity in your home with a hygrometer, an inexpensive gadget available at hardware stores. If you get higher than 50 percent humidity, you may be inviting mildew, mold and dust mites.

6. **Wash bedding in hot water.** Washing sheets, pillows and blankets in hot water—at least 130 degrees—will kill dust mites and eggs.

7. **Test for radon.** Radon is a radioactive gas that occurs naturally in soil. It's the second-leading cause of lung cancer and the No. 1 cause of lung cancer among nonsmokers,[58] and it can creep into your home through cracks. Checking radon levels is easy and inexpensive with tests you can buy at a hardware store or by hiring a professional. If levels are at 4 pCi/L or higher, the problem needs to be addressed. Learn more about radon mitigation at the EPA's website: *www.epa.gov/radon/radontest.html.*

8. **Keep up your carbon monoxide detectors.** Carbon monoxide is an invisible, odorless gas that can be fatal in minutes. Lower levels of carbon monoxide can lead to headaches, dizziness and fatigue, according to the EPA.[59] Carbon monoxide comes from a variety of sources, including poorly ventilated gas stoves, leaking furnaces, car exhaust and tobacco smoke, and it can accumulate indoors. Carbon monoxide detectors can be purchased at hardware stores. They should be placed in or near bedrooms, and batteries should be checked regularly. It's also a good idea to hire a professional to

regularly inspect your heating system to ensure carbon monoxide doesn't become a problem.

9. **Maintain a no-shoes-in-the-house policy.**

10. **Dust regularly.** Use slightly damp cloth to avoid whipping up more dust into the air. Use a touch of water or a natural product to dust (see the cleaning section for more details), not an aerosol spray made of chemicals. Dusting once a week is ideal, but if that's not realistic, just make a point to do it as regularly as possible. Don't forget about hard-to-reach places, like above kitchen cabinets, where a vacuum might help with the job.

11. **Sweep, vacuum and mop regularly.** Use a vacuum with a HEPA filter to grab the smallest of particles off your floors. Mop using water or other natural ingredients, such as vinegar.

12. **Use household plants to clean the air.** It's amazing how well nature helps us out if we let it—certain plants naturally filter the air. NASA studied some of the best plants for removing all kinds of unhealthy substances: formaldehyde, ammonia, acetate, benzene and more. Some of the top cleaners include devil's ivy, peace lilies, Pleomele, gerbera daisies, Sansevieria trifasciata (snake plant), English ivy, spider plants, philodendrons, chrysanthemums and red-edged dracaena. Place these plants throughout your home. See "How to Grow Fresh Air: 50 House Plants that Purify Your Home or Office," by B.C. Wolverton.

13. **Be aware of those household plants that can be allergens or irritants.** Plants that pollinate in winter can be a problem for some people—ask a knowledgeable employee at a plant store about which plants are less likely to be irritating. You'll also want to keep an eye out to ensure mildew and mold don't start growing in or underneath plants. Keep in mind that some plants are dangerous when ingested, so if you have babies or pets around, make sure to keep those plants out of reach.

14. **Hire a building biologist** to evaluate the air quality in your home.

KITCHEN

· · · · · · ·

"I think careful cooking is love, don't you? The loveliest thing you can cook for someone who's close to you is about as nice a valentine as you can give."

— JULIA CHILD

The products we use to store, prepare and cook food can leach undesirable chemicals into meals. But not to worry—choosing safer options for the kitchen is easy. See the resources on page 95.

1. **Don't use Teflon or nonstick pans, which are often coated in perflourinated chemicals (PFCs). Instead, choose stainless steel, anodized aluminum, copper-coated, cast iron or enamel-coated iron.** With a little practice, you can learn to cook on these materials without sticking food and major cleanups—although they might take a little more effort to clean than nonstick pans. If you can't replace your nonstick pan, use the fan when you cook with it and set your stove or oven to the lowest possible temperature that will work for your cooking and baking needs.

2. **Avoid plastic—period—but especially plastic marked No. 3 or No. 7. Choose glass, stainless steel, ceramic or porcelain instead.** Invest in items such as glass food-storage containers, stainless steel measuring cups, and wood or metal cooking and baking utensils. They might cost more initially, but they're a good investment. Not only will glass, stainless steel, ceramic,

etc., probably outlast plastic (which gets cracked, scratched and warped), but also natural products will keep you and your family healthier—plastic is associated with many health issues.

The problems start at the molecular level. Plastic is made from petroleum, and the manufacturing of plastic releases toxic chemicals into the environment. In addition, plastics can take a millennium or more to break down, and they cause environmental (and then health) damage in the meantime. A more direct issue with plastics is that they break down—especially when heated—and can release harmful chemicals into food and drinks.

Some plastic contains bisphenol a (BPA), a known endocrine-disrupting chemical that's used to harden plastics. BPA leaches out of products and into food, drinks and people's bodies. Studies have found links between BPA exposure and myriad health issues, including behavioral changes, cancer, cardiovascular disease, diabetes, early puberty, male and female infertility and obesity.[60] Plastics marked with No. 1, 2, 4 or 5 don't have BPA, so they're a better choice. See the Environmental Working Group's Guide to BPA, at *www.ewg.org/bpa*.

Another problem with some plastics is polyvinyl chloride (PVC), which is widely used and extremely toxic. It's found in baby bibs, table cloths, disposable food and beverage bottles, and plastic food wrapping. When PVC is used in a soft plastic, it's made with phthalates. Remember, phthalates are a class of chemicals that can increase the risk for asthma and allergies, negatively impact behavior and mood, cause delayed sexual development in baby boys and damage DNA in sperm.[61][62][63][64]

3. **Buy foods that use phthalate-free packaging.** Many grocery store meats and cheeses are wrapped in plastics that contain phthalates. Find out about the brands you're buying, and if needed, switch to a company using phthalate-free wrapping.

4. **If you use a plastic wrap for food storage, find one that states it does not use PVC and that uses LDPE plastic instead.** Plastic wrap often touches food, so the chemicals contained in the wrap can migrate into the food. Nobody wants a sprinkling of PVC atop his or her meal. Unlike PVC, low-density polyethylene plastic

KITCHEN 41

(LDPE) is not currently known to have harmful additives. No matter what plastic wrap you use, try to keep it from directly touching your food.

5. **Avoid products with antibacterial claims.** Disinfect with vinegar and hydrogen peroxide. Antibacterial cutting boards and other products are often made with the hormone-disrupting chemical triclosan.[65] Instead, you can disinfect by simply wetting a paper towel with vinegar and wiping down the surface. Then wet another paper towel with hydrogen peroxide and wipe it down again.

6. **Choose canned goods that are BPA free.** BPA is often used to line metal food cans, and it can leach out from the lining into the food.

7. **Instead of plastic, use glass canning jars for food storage.** At about $1 apiece or less, these jars are versatile and long lasting, and they come in many sizes. When you get home from grocery shopping, remove dried foods—such as flour, chocolate, beans, rice and other bulk items—from their packages and pour them into glass jars. These foods keep well in a pantry, where you can easily see what's in the jar and how much is left. The jars work well for storing leftovers too, and they're easy to toss into a dishwasher for cleaning. If you buy multiple sets of these jars, always choose ones with the same width for the lids so you don't have to sort through your lids to find the right match.

8. **Instead of plastic bags, choose reusable bags that are free of BPA, phthalates and PVC.** Ideally, look for reusable, washable bags made of organic cotton. Find these in natural food stores or online.

9. **Ditch the plastic water bottles, baby bottles and sippy cups.** Use stainless steel or glass options instead.

10. **If you want plastic for toddler or children's dishes, look for products free of BPA, phthalates and melamine.** The brand Green Toys has a nice line called Green Eats that meets these qualifications and are affordable. *www.greentoys.com/greeneats*

FURNITURE

• • • • • • •

"I consider that a man's brain originally is like a little empty attic, and you have to stock it with such furniture as you choose."

—ARTHUR CONAN DOYLE

Selecting furniture can be quite a process. But if you're working to limit your household exposure to VOCs, flame retardants and carcinogens, your efforts to create a healthy home will narrow down your options, and in this way, make shopping easier. Remember to apply these tips when shopping for children's furniture too.

1. **Choose natural fibers,** such as cotton, linen, wool, bamboo or silk, and avoid plastic, vinyl and foam.

2. **Buy organic fabrics when possible.** Cotton is one of the dirtiest crops around—it's usually heavily doused in pesticides, and the pesticides it uses are particularly hazardous. Skip the chemicals and choose an organic fabric for your health.

3. **Research whether, and what, flame retardants are used.** Upholstered furniture, especially items made with polyurethane foam, often contains chemical flame retardants. The older an item is (unless it's made before 1975 when flame retardant laws were widely adopted), the more the materials break down and easily let chemicals loose.

Furniture made with only polyester, down or wool is unlikely to contain chemical flame retardants. Also, due to a change in California law, more flame-retardant free options are becoming available across the country. Suppliers that offer furniture that's free of added flame retardants include: Cisco Home (*www.ciscohome.net*), Eco-Terric (*www.eco-terric.com*), EcoBalanza (*www.greenerlifestyles.com*), Ekla Home (*www.eklahome.com*), Furnature (*www.furnature.com*), GreenSofas (*www.greensofas.com*), Viesso (*www.viesso.com*) and The Futon Shop (*www.thefutonshop.com*). There are some additional suppliers available outside California, although you might need to request flame-retardant free from some of these: Corinthian (*www.corinthianfurn.com*), Drexel Heritage (*www.drexelheritage.com*), EcoSelect (*www.ecoselectfurniture.com*), Endicott Home (*www.condosofa.com*) and LEE Industries (*www.leeindustries.com*).

The Center for Environmental Health lists brands that make flame retardant-free furniture and products: *www.ceh.org/campaigns/flame-retardants/ceh-action/finding-safer-products/*.

4. **Note that covering furniture, for example with a slipcover, doesn't eliminate chemicals from migrating.** The chemicals aren't usually bound, which means they make their way out of original materials and through covers.

5. **Avoid stain-resistant coatings that may be added to your furniture.** Shop for furniture that doesn't use these coatings. Sometimes you can ask the manufacturer to skip that finishing step.

6. **Choose solid wood** and avoid fiberboard, particleboard and pressed wood.

7. **Look for a safe and natural wood finish**, that is, a water-based finish or one that uses certain plant oils.

8. **Remember to consider the materials used in shades, blinds and curtains.** Many window coverings, and especially those marketed as light blocking, use a fabric that contains plastics, including PVC, and chemical residues. These materials can off-gas and

release VOCs, especially when they heat up from sunlight. Look for curtains made of 100 percent cotton, bamboo, hemp, linen or solid wood. A darker, thick natural fabric will help block the light. Make your own to save money and have better control over the fabric and materials.

9. **Remember that children's furniture is no exception and can also contain chemicals and flame retardants.** In 2013, the Center for Environmental Health, with support from Alliance for a Healthy Tomorrow, submitted children's furniture items from major retailers across several states for independent testing. The results showed that four flame retardant chemicals were present in 38 of the 42 items tested. The chemicals found have been linked to cancer, hormone disruption, infertility and other health problems.[66]

ELECTRONICS

....

"Water, air, and cleanness are the chief articles in my pharmacy."
—NAPOLEON BONAPARTE

Most electronics contain flame retardant chemicals, either inside the product or in the plastic case surrounding the product. When the electronics heat up during use, they're even more likely to emit these chemicals into the air you breathe.

1. **Buy electronics from companies that do not use PBDE flame retardants.** Some manufacturers have pledged to avoid this dangerous class of chemicals. According to the Environmental Working Group, the following companies have publicly stated their commitment to phasing out PBDEs: Acer, Apple, Eizo Nanao, LG Electronics, Lenovo, Matsushita, Microsoft, Nokia, Phillips, Samsung, Sharp, Sony-Ericsson, and Toshiba.[67] Before buying a new product, ask whether PBDEs are used and choose one that is free of PBDEs.

2. **Avoid standing next to printers and copy machines while they're in use.** The closer you are, the more chemicals and emissions you're breathing in. If possible, open a window while printing and copying are underway, and leave the room for a bit.

MATTRESSES AND BEDDING

. . . .

"As you make your bed, so you must lie in it."
—DANIEL J. BOORSTIN

People (should) spend about one-third of their life sleeping. That means our beds get a lot of use. As we breathe and lie in bed, the materials in our mattresses have plenty of time to impact our health. Beds are notorious for containing toxic materials, including chemical flame retardants, vinyl, PVCs, antimony and other chemical finishes. Sleep experts say some people find that greening up their bedrooms—thereby reducing chemical exposure and VOCs—leads to more restful sleep.

1. **Get to know some of the top truly healthy mattress brands,** including Naturepedic, Savvy Rest, European Sleep Works, Green Sleep, Shepherd's Dream and Soaring Heart Natural Bed Company.

2. **Avoid polyurethane foam, vinyl and synthetic latex. Choose mattresses made of cotton, wool, or the plant-based materials natural latex, coconut husk, mohair, kapok and buckwheat.** Polyurethane foam, which is also in memory foam and soy foam, is often the main material of choice for mattresses. It can contain many chemicals, including formaldehyde, benzene and toluene, and it can emit VOCs into your home. Other things to watch out for in most mattresses: Vinyl is made with vinyl chloride monomer, a known carcinogen[68] and synthetic latex may emit VOCs.

   With natural mattresses, including those made with organic

cotton or wool, you won't have to worry about years of inhaling toxic chemicals as they off-gas. Wool can also naturally deter stains, moisture, mites and bacteria.

3. **Avoid mattresses with chemical flame retardants in any part of their materials or coverings and opt for those that use wool or hydrated silica instead.** Choose mattresses that use wool, a natural flame retardant, or hydrated silica, another safer choice.

4. **Shop for mattresses from companies that discloses all their materials online or that will disclose their materials if you request them.** At the time of Clean and Healthy New York's research for "The Mattress Matters" report, only two companies, Naturepedic and Soaring Heart Natural Bed Co., fully disclosed on their websites all the chemicals and materials they used to make their mattresses. Nearly 40 percent of the manufacturers refused to fully disclose the materials they used. Most often, they refused information about how they make mattresses flame resistant, waterproof or antimicrobial.[69]

5. **Know that babies and children's mattresses often contain potentially harmful chemical flame retardants.** Juvenile mattresses made from polyurethane foam likely contain these chemicals. Opt for children's mattresses that use wool or hydrated silica as the flame retardant.

6. **Avoid bedding, especially for babies and children, that has vinyl and PVC plastic.** These materials frequently cover mattresses for babies and kids, and they can emit fumes that are inhaled all night long. PVC is a highly toxic plastic that contains phthalates, a class of hormone-disrupting chemicals that have been shown to impact sexual development;[70] increase the risk for allergy and asthma; negatively affect behavior; impair sperm quality, reproductive hormone levels and thyroid function;[71] and damage DNA in men's sperm.[72]

7. **When you need to prevent leaks and accidents, buy wool mattress pads instead of waterproof plastic pads.** Wool natu-

rally resists moisture without the chemical treatment. There are many options for baby- and kid-sized wool mattress pads.

8. **Take your time shopping for a mattress for babies and children.** Their developing brains and bodies are more susceptible to the harmful effects of chemical exposure. They also spend much more time asleep than adults. One report from Clean and Healthy New York found that 72 percent of crib mattresses surveyed used one or more chemicals of concern, including antimony, vinyl, polyurethane foam and other VOCs.[73] If you have a little one, it's worth your time to download "The Mattress Matters" report from Clean and Healthy New York: *www.media.wix.com/ugd/a2c2a6_7d59219c7ef3023b5472ef84017c6ab7.pdf*

9. **Choose untreated organic mattresses when possible.**

10. **Consider futons for a more affordable option.** Many futon mattresses are at least free of polyurethane foam and instead use cotton or wool. The cotton or wool mattresses are frequently treated with boric acid, a less toxic flame retardant. Futon mattresses with enough wool can meet flame retardant standards without the boric acid and will probably be cheaper than a traditional wool mattress. Futon mattresses are a great option for kids. Adults might find they're comfortable as well, but it's best to test them out first. Some futon shops will make mattresses without flame retardants if you have a doctor's note about the need to avoid chemicals.

11. **Be aware of misleading claims.** A mattress might include one layer of organic cotton—attracting health- and eco-conscious consumers—but still use plenty of other harmful materials.

12. **Skip box springs and choose a bed frame that uses solid-wood slats.** Box springs are more likely to use synthetic materials. Skip the unknown and opt for solid-wood platform beds..

LINENS AND BATHROOM

. . . .

"There must be quite a few things that a hot bath won't cure, but I don't know many of them."
—SYLVIA PLATH

As you snuggle up under your blankets at night or dry off with a soft towel after a shower, the last thing you want to think about is being covered in a cocoon of chemicals. Unfortunately, many linens today are made with synthetic materials and contain chemical finishes and dyes that could be absorbed through the skin or inhaled when you breathe. Better choices are easy to find.

1. **For sheets, blankets, pillows, mattress toppers and towels, choose natural materials,** such as cotton, linen, hemp, bamboo, silk, wool, kapok or buckwheat. Skip vinyl, polyester and other synthetic fabrics. When you learn what synthetic materials are made of, it doesn't sound too cozy. Polyester, for instance, is made out of petroleum and other chemicals. Sticking with natural materials for your linens will minimize your exposure to chemicals and off-gassing materials.

2. **Choose unbleached, untreated, organic fabrics when possible.**

3. **Buy products that use eco-friendly or "low-impact" dyes.**

4. **Avoid products that say they're stain-resistant, water-resistant, no-iron or "easy care."** These are likely to contain harmful chemicals. Wool, however, is naturally water-resistant.

5. **Skip products that say they're antibacterial.** Keep linens clean by washing them in water that's 130 degrees or hotter.

6. **Wash linens before using them.**

7. **Choose shower curtains made from natural materials, such as hemp or cotton.** Skip the plastic. And if you can't spend the money on a natural fabric curtain or liner, choose a plastic curtain that states it's PVC free. Polyvinyl chloride (PVC) plastic is made with numerous toxic chemicals that let off VOCs into the air. One report showed that over a period of 28 days, new shower curtains emitted 108 VOCs, including phthalates, possible carcinogens and other chemicals known to affect the central nervous system, reproductive system, immune system, liver, kidneys and skin. The researchers found VOCs still lingering from the curtains after four weeks. According to the report, "seven of the chemicals released by the shower curtain are classified as hazardous air pollutants by the United States Environmental Protection Agency (EPA) under the Clean Air Act."[74] See *http://chej.org/campaigns/pvc/resources/shower-curtain-report/*

PAINT

. . . .

"When I judge art, I take my painting and put it next to a God made object like a tree or flower. If it clashes, it is not art."
—PAUL CEZANNE

A big paint project or a little touchup here and there can expose you and your household to chemicals you're better off avoiding. Be informed next time you bust out those brushes.

1. **Choose paint with no VOCs (or at least low VOCs).** Everyone knows the scent of fresh paint. What everyone might not know is that with every sniff, you're smelling all the chemicals you're simultaneously inhaling. And those chemicals linger beyond the time when your nose can detect them. Keep your air clear of VOCs by choosing a no-VOC paint. Look for products certified by GREENGUARD or Green Seal, or search for no-VOC options on these organizations' websites. If you decide you must go with a low-VOC option instead of no-VOC, do some quick research: Look on the paint can for where VOC grams per liter are listed and choose the one with the smallest number.

2. **Look for biocide-free paint.** Chemical biocides, which include pesticides and antimicrobials, are often added to paint. Avoid these toxic preservatives by choosing paint that is free of biocides.

3. **Avoid paint with NPEs (nonylphenol ethoxylates).** These chemicals mimic the human hormone estrogen, and they're extremely toxic to aquatic life. One report found that most household paints contain NPEs.[75]

4. **Use truly natural paints.** It's ideal to choose mineral, lime, clay or milk paints that use natural ingredients such as linseed oil, soy oil, beeswax or plant dye.

5. **Avoid wallpaper and vinyl.** Choose natural wall coverings, such as rice paper, cork, jute, bamboo, arrowroot or raffia. Many wallpapers use toxic glues and chemicals that off-gas.

6. **Be aware of lead if any parts of your home might have been painted before 1978.** Before you make changes to your walls or start to remodel, have your walls, windowsills and doors tested for lead paint, which can peel off, crack, get into household dust or be inhaled. Be sure to clean up paint chips immediately and regularly dust windowsills or door frames that are coated in lead paint. Never try to sand or remove lead paint yourself—it's extremely dangerous for you and anyone else living in your home. Instead, hire a professional who's been certified for lead-based paint removal by the EPA or by your state's agency.

7. **Use care when sanding.** Even if you already know no lead is in any of the layers of paint on your walls, other harmful chemicals might be, and they can be exposed in a big way when you sand. Be sure to wear proper eye and respiratory protection, ventilate the room, open windows and keep everyone who isn't working on the project out of the house. Clean up dust quickly and thoroughly.

FLOORS AND RUGS

• • • • • • •

"When you dance, your purpose is not to get to a certain place on the floor. It's to enjoy each step along the way."

—WAYNE DYER

Keep your chemical exposure from flooring to a minimum by becoming an informed consumer and establishing some easy, healthy habits.

1. **Maintain a no-shoes-in-the-house rule** (this is even more important if you have babies or children in your home).

2. **Avoid carpet or replace it when you can.** Carpet is often made of all kinds of harmful substances that are used in its fibers or backing materials, and it often contains hazardous stain-proofing chemicals and dyes. Carpet can off-gas VOCs for years. Plus, carpet cushion often contains flame retardant chemicals. On top of that, anything in a home—dust, dust mites, dander, pesticides, lead, bacteria, mold and allergens—gets easily buried and trapped in carpet.

3. **For deep carpet cleaning, look for a "green" and water-based system.** Newer technologies mean that water alone can go a long way in cleaning your carpets and rugs. Skip the chemicals and harsh detergents by finding a cleaner that relies on water-based technologies with only truly natural soaps. Check out the ingredi-

ents list for yourself to be sure. One water-based option is *www.zerorez.com*

4. **If you put in new carpet, choose a natural wool, natural rubber, fiber or felt pad under the carpet instead of a bonded carpet cushion,** which likely contains flame retardants. More than 85 percent of the carpet cushion made in the United States is made with bonded polyurethane carpet cushion, which usually contains flame retardants.

5. **Research chemical finishes on all rugs, carpets and their backing or cushions to avoid such treatments as stain repellants, insect repellants or flame retardants.** Even natural rugs might be coated with these chemicals.

6. **If you put in new carpet, look for recycled, low- or no-VOC carpets that aren't glued to the floor.** Carpet tiles are a great option, but check with the manufacturer to ensure the tiles are free of PVC. Once the carpet is installed, keep babies and children off it as long as you can.

7. **If you have carpet,** regularly steam clean your carpet (with a water-based, non-chemical cleaning process) and use a HEPA filter vacuum.

8. **Buy rugs that are made of natural fibers,** such as jute, bamboo, wool, cotton seagrass, coir or sisal. Avoid rugs with a glued-on rubber backing. These natural fibers won't emit harmful chemicals. Look for a backing or pad that also uses a natural material, including wool, jute or natural latex. Ideally, the backing should be sewed on, not glued.

9. **Choose organic wool and cotton.** This will further limit your exposure to pesticides used in growing or treating the materials, as well as to harsh chemical finishing treatments.

10. **Buy rugs that are washable.**

11. **Skip vinyl, linoleum and imitation wood floors.** Choose flooring made from natural materials: solid wood, bamboo, natural cork, stone, natural tile or natural linoleum (which is made from materials such as linseed oil, limestone dust and jute). These natural materials won't off-gas dangerous VOCs, unlike carpet, vinyl and linoleum. They'll also likely last longer and look nicer, perhaps saving money in the long run.

12. **Be aware of the glues and finishes in your floors.** Glues and stains often use unhealthy chemicals. Look for bamboo that's laid without glue and without adhesives. Finish hardwood floors with a water-based varnish certified by Green Seal or GREENGUARD.

CLEANING PRODUCTS

• • • • • • •

"Life is denied by lack of attention, whether it be to cleaning windows or trying to write a masterpiece."
—NADIA BOULANGER

It's ironic—and sad—that most of the cleaning products on the market today make homes dirtier, as they leave a film of unhealthy chemicals and release VOCs into the air. Many commonly used cleaning ingredients are linked with health conditions, including asthma, cancer and reproductive problems. The majority of the ingredients used in cleaning products aren't even required to be listed on the label. Fortunately, there are easy ways to clean your home with healthy products.

1. **Opt for truly natural products, including those certified by Green Seal or EcoLogo, or make your own—it's easy and can save a lot of money.** People used homemade products for most of human history, and they work well. Find easy and effective cleaning recipes online and in books. Here are some common natural cleaning ingredients:
   - **White vinegar** kills mold and bacteria, cuts wax and grease buildup and helps dissolve mineral buildup, soap scum, water spots and rust. Vinegar is a natural disinfectant that works great for cleaning floors or mixed in with a general-purpose cleaning solution.

- **Baking soda** neutralizes minerals, helps soap clean better, absorbs odors and works great to clean sinks and tubs. Baking soda also effectively cleans ovens, toilets and showers.
- **Olive oil** can be used to polish furniture.
- **Lemon juice** removes stains, is a mild bleaching agent and fights mineral scum.
- **Essential oils** often contain natural cleaning properties. For example, lavender is antiviral, antibacterial and antifungal. Cinnamon is antiviral, and thyme is antibacterial. Essential oils are made using the oil of the plant they come from. They're often extracted from a plant through a distillation process, leading to a concentrated form of natural oil.
- **Hydrogen peroxide** is a natural disinfectant and bleaching agent that's also antimicrobial.
- **Castile soaps** are mild and versatile soaps made with olive oil. They're often used in homemade general-purpose solutions, scrubbing solutions and floor cleaners.

2. **Use the Environmental Working Group's cleaning products database to find safer products.** Here you can search for more than 2,000 products and see how they rank for health: *www.ewg.org/guides/cleaners*.

3. **Be aware that most cleaning products use harmful chemicals, including known carcinogens, hormone-disrupting chemicals and neurotoxins.** The children of women who work as custodians or cleaners have "significantly elevated risks of birth defects," according to a 2010 study from the New York State Department of Health.[76]

    One air pollution study by the Environmental Working Group examined 21 products commonly used to clean schools. It found that the products released a large range of pollutants, including those linked to asthma, cancer, reproductive toxicity, hormone disruption and neurotoxicity. According to the report, "some of the worst offenders are in products also commonly used in the home." For example, the 2009 study showed that at the time Comet Disinfectant Cleanser Powder emitted 146 chemicals, and Febreze Air Effects released 89 air contaminants.[77] Along those lines, children born into homes that used more chemical products were more likely to experience respiratory problems.[78] Another study concluded that "[f]requent use of common household cleaning sprays may be an important risk factor for adult asthma."[79]

4. **Don't be fooled by marketing and labels.** Some products are labeled as "non-toxic," "natural," "green" and "biodegradable" but still use some unhealthy chemicals.

5. **Avoid chemical products with antibacterial claims.**

6. **Skip products with fragrance.** Fragrance often contains dangerous unlisted chemicals, including phthalates, which are hormone-disrupting chemicals that have been shown to impact sexual development;[80] increase the risk for allergy and asthma; negatively affect behavior; impair sperm quality, reproductive hormone levels and thyroid function;[81] and damage DNA in sperm.[82]

7. **Avoid cleaning products with dyes.** Dyes can contain a host of harmful chemicals and they're unnecessary.

8. **Skip aerosol sprays.** Instead, use a spray bottle for homemade recipes. The tiny particles from aerosols hang in the air longer than you'd expect and can contribute to health problems.

9. **Become an advocate for healthier cleaning products in your child's school.** One resource that can come in handy is the Green Cleaning for Healthy Schools Toolkit, at *www.cleaningforhealthyschools.org*.

10. **Avoid products with these chemicals or ingredients:** 2-butoxyethanol, ethylene glycol monobutyl ether and other glycol ethers; alkylphenol ethoxylates, such as nonyl- and octylphenol ethoxylate, or non- and octoxynols; dye; ethanoloamines, such as mono-, di- and tri-ethanolamine; fragrance; pine or citrus oil (which can react with ozone to form formaldehyde); and quaternary ammonium compounds, such as alkyl dimethyl benzyl ammonium chlo-

ride (ADBAC), benzalkonium chloride and didecyl dimethyl benzyl ammonium chloride.[83]

11. **Be aware of and avoid formaldehyde and formaldehyde-releasing ingredients.** Numerous ingredients used in cleaning products release formaldehyde, a known carcinogen. Among them are DMDM hydantoin (Glydant), bronopol (2-bromo-2-nitropropane-1,3-diol), quaternium-15, imidazolidinyl urea, diazolidinyl urea, hydroxymethylglycinate and hexahydro-1,3,5-tris (2-hydroxethyl)-S-triazine (Grotan).[84]

LAUNDRY

• • • • • • •

"We should all do what, in the long run, gives us joy, even if it is only picking grapes or sorting the laundry."
—E.B. WHITE

Much like household cleaning products, laundry detergents and treatments often use harsh chemicals that are bad for you and the environment. Your clothes sit right on your skin, so it's smart to be thoughtful about what you use for laundering.

1. **Make your own laundry detergent.** It's easy and can save money. A search online will bring up many recipes for liquid or powder detergents. The recipes often combine a few common ingredients, such as castile soap, baking soda, super washing soda (which is similar to baking soda but stronger), and essential oils (for people who want some natural fragrance). You can quickly make big batches of these homemade detergents.

2. **If DIY isn't your thing, buy truly natural products, such as those certified by Green Seal or EcoLogo.** Choose detergents that use plant- or vegetable-based ingredients. (Most products are petroleum-based). Look for products that are also biodegradable and free of phosphates. When laundry chemicals are rinsed down the drain, they end up in our lakes, streams and waterways. Many don't biodegrade, thereby polluting water supplies and harming fish, wildlife and people.

3. **Use the Environmental Working Group's website** that ranks laundry products. See *www.ewg.org/guides/categories/9-Laundry*.

4. **Know the problems with most detergent and laundry products.** These often contain petroleum products, optical brighteners, chlorine bleach, phenols, chemical surfactants, ammonia, and synthetic and toxic fragrances and dyes. Commonly used laundry chemicals are linked to cancer, hormone disruption, neurological and reproductive effects and more.

5. **Instead of a chemical fabric softener, add to the rinse cycle one-half cup of baking soda or one-fourth cup white distilled vinegar.**

6. **Skip dryer sheets,** which often contain nasty chemicals. Find safer alternatives. Look for reusable, cloth-based dryer sheets and wool dryer balls, available at eco-conscious stores, natural food stores and online.

7. **Avoid chlorine bleach.** Use hydrogen peroxide, vinegar or lemon juice to help remove stains. Chlorine bleach is a highly caustic chemical that can cause skin, eye, nose and respiratory irritation. It's also terrible for the environment, even at low levels. Instead, use one of the many natural stain removers easily at your disposal. For instance, spray stained collars with white distilled vinegar, let it sit for a bit and then toss the shirts into the wash.

8. **Naturally brighten fabrics with the sun.** Hanging clothes or linens out in the sun will naturally brighten them. Just avoid putting out dark fabrics on a sunny day, as they might fade. As an added bonus, hanging clothes out to dry can make them last longer because they're not getting tumbled around in high heat as much.

9. **Don't dry clean, or at least use a green dry cleaner.** Choose fabrics that don't require dry cleaning. If you already have some pieces that require it, find a green cleaner that doesn't use PERC, also called tetrachloroethylene or perchloroethylene. According to the EPA, studies show that people who wear dry-cleaned clothes

or who have dry-cleaned items in their homes breathe in low levels of PERC.[85] In addition, PERC can accumulate in the body, where it's stored in fat. Further, women who are exposed to this chemical have an increased risk for breast cancer.[86] A healthier option is a dry cleaner that uses a process known as wet cleaning, CO2 cleaning or GreenEarth, which cleans with liquid silicone, which is basically liquefied sand.

AIR FRESHENERS AND CANDLES

∙ ∙ ∙ ∙ ∙ ∙ ∙

*"A true poet does not bother to be poetical.
Nor does a nursery gardener scent his roses."*
—JEAN COCTEAU

Air fresheners are inaccurately named—most of them emit VOCs, phthalates and other harmful ingredients, making air more polluted. And they certainly don't clean the air; they just cover up odors with a concoction of chemicals. That cozy glow of a candle also often lets off harmful chemicals and pollutants into your home. Better choices are readily available.

1. **Skip chemical air fresheners and paraffin candles and be aware of their hazards.** Most emit harmful chemicals, including VOCs and phthalates, even when they say they're "natural" or "unscented" or don't use dyes.

2. **Use the Environmental Working Group's air freshener guide** to see how products rank: *www.ewg.org/guides/subcategories/ 1-AirFreshener*

3. **Clean your air naturally with houseplants.** As previously mentioned, certain plants naturally filter your air, and NASA studied some of the best ones for doing the job. These plants remove all kinds of unhealthy products: formaldehyde, ammonia, acetate, benzene and more. Some of the top cleaners include

devil's ivy, peace lilies, Pleomele, gerbera daisies, Sansevieria trifasciata (snake plant), English ivy, spider plants, philodendrons, chrysanthemums and red-edged dracaena. Place these plants and others throughout your home. See the book "How to Grow Fresh Air: 50 House Plants that Purify Your Home or Office" by B.C. Wolverton for more details.

4. **Clean your air with baking soda, a natural deodorizer and air freshener.** There are many options here, including:
   1. Fill glass canning jars with some baking soda and a few drops of a pure essential oil (such as lavender, tea tree or peppermint). Remove the main lid from the jar top and replace it with some pretty paper, then pop several small holes in the paper and place it back in the lid ring. Set the jars in your bathroom, kitchen or anywhere that could use some regular freshening. Give the jar a little shake every now and then.
   2. Boil two cups of water. Add a teaspoon of baking soda and mix until dissolved, then add a teaspoon of lemon juice and mix. Pour the solution into a spray bottle and spritz it into the air as needed.

5. **Infuse fragrance into the air naturally with essential oils or by boiling certain herbs, spices or plants.** A couple methods include:
   1. Simmer cinnamon, cloves, citrus peel or flower petals on the stovetop for a bit.
   2. Add several drops of a pure essential oil into distilled water, mix and pour into a spray bottle. Shake before spritzing.

6. **Skip paraffin candles and be aware of their hazards.** Paraffin candles, derived from petroleum, are the most common and inexpensive type of candle. According to the EPA, they emit harmful chemicals, including formaldehyde, acetaldehyde and acrolein.[87]

7. **Buy 100 percent beeswax candles.** Some might have misleading labels and say they use "pure beeswax," but that doesn't mean the candle is 100 percent beeswax. Soy candles also likely burn cleaner than paraffin, but some critics say soy also has its downfalls.

8. **Beware of lead in candle wicks.** Lead is sometimes found in the wicks of candles made outside the U.S. When the candle burns, it releases lead into the air, where it's readily inhaled.

TOYS AND PRODUCTS FOR BABIES AND CHILDREN

• • • • • • •

"Our inventions are wont to be pretty toys, which distract our attention from serious things. They are but improved means to an unimproved end."
—HENRY DAVID THOREAU

It's especially important that the materials used for babies' and children's toys are safe, as little ones are constantly touching and sucking on these products. Harmful chemicals more easily damage their small but rapidly developing brains and bodies. And because youngsters' detoxification systems are less mature, it's harder for their bodies to clean out pollutants.

Toys and children's products commonly contain harmful substances, including carcinogens, lead, flame retardants, arsenic, PVC and hormone-disrupting chemicals. Those substances can slough off or evaporate, and they can be ingested when the item is sucked on or chewed.

The American Academy of Pediatrics in 2011 issued a policy statement calling for better protection of pregnant women and children from chemicals: "As children grow and mature, their bodies may be especially vulnerable to certain chemical exposures during critical windows of development. Neurologic and endocrine systems have demonstrated particular sensitivity to environmental toxicants at certain stages of growth." The academy also says, "A growing body of research indicates potential harm to child health from a range of chemical substances."[88]

Finding toys that are safe might cost a little more because plastic is about as cheap as you can get, but you can't put a price on your child's health and future. Buy fewer but better-quality toys to offset the higher cost of natural materials. As an added bonus, this will keep your home less cluttered and give it a more peaceful feel than a room overflowing with junky plastic toys. Plus, toys made of high-quality, natural materials will outlast plastic and are more likely to be treasured and passed on for generations.

1. **Get to know the brands that make safer, healthier toys,** including Plan Toys, Under the Nile, MiYim, Apple Park, Haba and Green Toys. You can buy direct from some of their websites. Additional sites that sell various brands of healthier toys include www.novanatural.com, www.oompa.com, www.ourgreenhouse.com, www.palumba.com, www.peapods.com, www.planethappytoys.com, www.rosiehippo.com and www.thewoodenwagon.com.

2. **Avoid plastic.** Many harmful ingredients are used in plastic toys, and babies and children take in those ingredients when they touch, chew, suck or mouth a toy.[89][90] Hazardous ingredients, such as the ones below, can also leach out and dust off from toys.
   - **Phthalates.** As previously mentioned, these hormone-disrupting chemicals have been shown to impact sexual development;[91] increase the risk for allergy and asthma; negatively affect behavior; impair sperm quality, reproductive hormone levels and thyroid function;[92] and damage DNA in sperm.[93] The U.S. government recently banned some types of phthalates from children's toys (and a few are banned only on an interim basis).[94] But that doesn't protect you from other potentially harmful phthalates or plastic toys manufactured before the ban.
   - **BPA.** The FDA banned this hormone-disrupting chemical from baby bottles and sippy cups in 2012.[95] But BPA is still found many other places, including toys. One report found BPA in 280 plastic toys.[96]
   - **PVC.** This substance, often used in plastic squeeze toys, is made from vinyl chloride, a carcinogen.[97] PVC in soft materials contains unhealthy chemicals, including chlorine, phthalates and BPA[98] and it migrates off products. You can identify it through the No. 3 symbol on the bottom of plastic.

3. **Choose solid wood in toys** and avoid brands that use pressed wood, particleboard or imitation wood.

4. **Look for truly safe paints and finishes, not just those that say "nontoxic."** Avoid the bath of chemicals by choosing products with natural finishes, such as linseed oil, walnut oil or beeswax, and paints that are water- or plant-based.

5. **Avoid foam,** which is used in many baby products, stuffed toys and children's furniture. Foam can contain many chemicals, including formaldehyde, benzene and toluene, and emit VOCs into your home. One study found that more than 80 percent of the baby products tested, including nursing pillows and changing pads, contained chemical flame retardants.[99]

   Opt for healthier toy brands, such as Under the Nile, which uses organic cotton stuffing for their soft toys and stuffed animals.

6. **Choose natural fibers.** Cotton, wool, linen and bamboo are safer choices than synthetic fabrics, such as polyester, acrylic, rayon, nylon and fleece.

7. **Buy organic products when possible, including children's stuffed animals.**

8. **Look for eco-friendly dyes or "low-impact" dyes.**

9. **For soft toys, such as bath toys or teething products, look for 100 percent natural rubber.**

10. **Look for safer art materials made from natural materials,** such as beeswax or soy, and paints that use vegetable-based dyes and pigments. Many art supplies are made from petroleum or use other petrochemicals, or they can emit harmful chemicals and VOCs. If your child's paint or markers smell, get rid of them. Some websites that sell safer brands of art supplies include *www.novanatural.com, www.oompa.com, www.ourgreenhouse.com, www.palumba.com, www.planethappytoys.com, www.rosie-hippo.com* and *www.thewoodenwagon.com*.

11. **See how thousands of toys rank for health** by searching for products at *www.HealthyStuff.org*.

12. **If you really want a plastic product, buy only plastic that has no PVC, phthalates or BPA and uses no external coatings.** Avoid plastic with the No. 3 on the bottom, as this indicates the product has PVC. High-density polyethylene (HDPE), which has the No. 2 recycling symbol, is considered a safer plastic than most. The brand Green Toys is one safer choice for plastic toys.

13. **Be leery about antique toys, hand-me-downs and garage-sale finds.** That generations-old toy might have sentimental value, but it's also much more likely to contain lead and other materials that are now banned or at least limited in toys today.

14. **Be aware of lead.** Lead levels are supposed to be limited in toys, but the chemical is still found regularly in levels above the federal limits. Most toys with lead are imported from countries that lack good control. However, one study of more than 1,500 children's toys found lead in 20 percent of the products, including toys manufactured in the U.S. More than 50 of the toys in the study contained lead levels above the federal recall standards for lead in paint.[100]

15. **Be aware of other harmful materials, including cadmium, mercury and arsenic.** A study of more than 1,500 toys found that 19 percent contained arsenic, 38 percent contained cadmium (a known carcinogen) and 4 percent contained mercury.[101]

16. **Skip the toy jewelry.** A study of more than 1,500 toys found that jewelry was five times more likely to contain high levels of lead than other products.[102] Another study of low-cost jewelry found that 59 percent of the products tested had a "high level of concern due to the presence of one or more hazardous chemicals detected at high levels."[103] Half of the items contained lead, one-third contained PVC, 7 percent contained brominated flame retardants and a handful contained cadmium.

17. **Skip kids' makeup and face paint.** A 2011 study of 31 products marketed to children showed that they all contained one or more hazardous materials, including arsenic, antimony, mercury and lead.[104] You can find natural face paint recipes online and make your own, which gives you complete control over the ingredients.

CLOTHES

. . . .

"Clothe yourselves with compassion, kindness, humility, gentleness and patience."
—COLOSSIANS 3:12

Your clothes sit against your skin (your largest organ) all day long—and so do any chemical treatments or coatings that have been used in manufacturing the clothes. Choose cleaner fabrics, and your whole body will breathe easier. Although it might cost more per item, you might find it refreshing to pare down your wardrobe to have fewer, but higher quality, pieces.

1. **Choose clothes made of natural fabrics,** including cotton, linen, silk, wool and cashmere. They likely contain fewer chemicals than synthetics.

2. **Whenever you can, avoid clothes made of synthetic fabrics,** such as acrylic, polyester, nylon, rayon and fleece. These are often derived from petroleum and plastics and are typically made with chemical treatments.

3. **Don't buy clothing that says it's stain resistant, wrinkle resistant, antibacterial, moth resistant or "no iron."** These clothes probably were produced using chemical treatments, such as perflorochemicals (PFCs).

4. **Buy untreated, organic clothing whenever possible** (GOTS certified products are a great choice). These items should be free of the chemicals used in clothing fibers and finishes.

5. **Be aware that some babies' and kids' pajamas contain chemical flame retardants.** Sleepwear for babies under 9 months old and pajamas that are tight fitting likely don't contain chemical flame retardants. Look for a tag that says something like, "For child's safety, garment should fit snugly. This garment is not flame resistant. Loose fitting garment is more likely to catch fire," or a tag that says the piece is "not intended as sleepwear." This type of language means the item is probably free of flame retardants.

    However, pajamas for babies 9 months old up to size 14 are required to pass certain flammability tests or to be "tight-fitting," according to the U.S. Consumer Product Safety Commission (CPSC) regulations.[105] The CPSC also requires children's sleepwear that's been treated with flame retardants to have a label that explains how to care for the item in order to maintain its flame resistance. Parents who wish to avoid flame retardant exposure can avoid buying clothes with this label.

    You can limit children's exposure to flame retardants by buying snug-fitting sleepwear that's certified organic. Or use tight-fitting regular clothes that are made of natural fibers such as cotton or wool for pajamas.

    Of course, it's always important to keep babies and kids a safe distance from open flames. And, it should go without saying that nobody should ever smoke near babies or children, for a whole host of health reasons.

    Aside from some pajamas for babies and kids, most clothing doesn't contain flame retardants.

6. **Wash clothes before you wear them.** This will help reduce your exposure to chemical residues that might have been used in the production process.

7. **Find organic clothes for babies and up** at www.underthenile.com, www.bamboosa.com, www.sagecreeknaturals.com, www.organicwearusa.com, www.ourgreenhouse.com, www.danishwool.com, www.purerest.com, www.novanatural.com.

PESTS

· · · · · · ·

"And all the insects ceased in honor of the moon."
—JACK KEROUAC

Nobody wants bugs, rodents or fungi around, but sprays, powders, balls, sticks and other synthetic methods of eliminating pests can affect human health too. Remember that the agents used to kill pests are designed to do just that: kill. Although people don't die from the amount of pesticide exposure that kills a pest, the exposure can still do harm, especially over time and when combined with multiple substances.

Products don't necessarily stay where they're sprayed or placed—they easily evaporate into the air you breathe. And without the sun and soil to help break them down, chemicals also last longer indoors than outdoors.

According to the EPA, "[O]ne study suggests that 80 percent of most people's exposure to pesticides occurs indoors, [and] preliminary research shows widespread presence of pesticide residues in homes."[106]

Health effects from pesticides, according to the EPA, can include "irritation to eye, nose and throat; damage to central nervous system and kidney; increased risk of cancer. Symptoms may include headache, dizziness, muscular weakness and nausea. Chronic exposure to some pesticides can result in damage to the liver, kidneys, endocrine and nervous system."[107]

Luckily, there's no need to contaminate your home with such chemicals—nature has a number of harmonious solutions for keeping things in order.

1. **Prevent the problem from happening in the first place with good housekeeping habits.** A dirty home is an invitation for critters and bugs. Maintain a no-shoes-in-the-house policy, dust regularly, sweep and vacuum regularly, repair leaks and cracks, clean up food and food scraps quickly and don't leave dirty dishes sitting out for long.

2. **Use or attract life forms in and around your home that naturally deter pests.** The herbs rosemary and catnip keep away mosquitoes, peppermint deters ants and mice, and ladybugs eat mites and aphids. Certain birds, including swallows, wrens and warblers, eat insect larvae and insect eggs. Placing a sprig of peppermint or lavender in the basement or kitchen can deter many pests.

3. **Use essential oils strategically.** Place a few drops of peppermint oil or citronella in cracks. Or, put the oils on cotton balls and leave the cotton balls in a problem pantry or closet.

4. **Use cedar chips, not mothballs, to repel moths.** Mothballs often contain a carcinogen.

5. **If needed, use integrated pest management (IPM) or biocides, also known as biopesticides, to naturally address a specific problem.** Biopesticides are made from plants, minerals, bacteria and other natural ingredients. According to the EPA, biopesticides "are usually inherently less toxic than conventional pesticides. Biopesticides generally affect only the target pest and closely related organisms, in contrast to broad spectrum, conventional pesticides that may affect organisms as different as birds, insects and mammals. Biopesticides often are effective in very small quantities and often decompose quickly, thereby resulting in lower exposures and largely avoiding the pollution problems caused by conventional pesticides."[108] Two resources for natural solutions are Pesticide Action Network's website, *www.panna.org*, and *www.beyondpesticides.org*.

LAWN AND GARDEN

· · · · · · ·

*"Earth provides enough to satisfy every man's
needs, but not every man's greed."*

—MAHATMA GANDHI

Pesticides and fertilizers seem like an easy way to keep a lawn or garden appearing nice and healthy. But a closer look shows that many kinds are actually damaging for vegetation and everyone in your home. Plus, chemical applications often lead to a domino effect, causing a lawn or garden to need more and more intervention and work.

Think of the grass in your yard as the tip of an iceberg. Below the grass are layers and layers of complex and interwoven forms of life: microbes, worms, fungi, nutrients and insects. Some are deeper down in the soil, and others hang out on the surface, but they all live pretty naturally in balance and rely on one another for good health. However, when chemicals are applied—whether pesticides, fertilizers, herbicides, insecticides or otherwise—that balance is thrown off as the product kills or harms multiple forms of life. That makes the soil, grass and plants more susceptible to disease and poor health.

Chemicals used outdoors are also readily tracked indoors, often on shoes or clothes. According to the President's Cancer Panel Report from 2010, Americans are exposed daily to numerous agricultural chemicals, partly through residential and commercial use. The report states, "[M]any of these chemicals have known or suspected carcinogenic or endocrine-disrupting properties. Pesticides (insecticides, herbicides, and fungicides) approved for use by the U.S. Environmental

Protection Agency (EPA) contain nearly 900 active ingredients, many of which are toxic."[109]

The report goes on to say that "[e]xposure to these chemicals has been linked to brain/central nervous system (CNS), breast, colon, lung, ovarian (female spouses), pancreatic, kidney, testicular and stomach cancers, as well as Hodgkin and non-Hodgkin lymphoma, multiple myeloma, and soft tissue sarcoma."

Children, the authors note, are most at risk for health effects from exposure. "Risks for childhood cancers are linked with parental pesticide exposure prior to conception, in utero exposure, and direct exposures throughout childhood. ... [L]eukemia rates are consistently elevated among children who grow up on farms, among children whose parents used pesticides in the home or garden, and among children of pesticide applicators."

Keep your lawn and garden—and yourself—truly healthy by skipping the chemical treatments and learning about organic lawn care.

1. **Pull weeds early in the season and use mulch annually instead of using herbicide.**

2. **Mow higher and leave grass clippings on the grass.** If your lawn looks like a minigolf venue, take note. Taller grass takes in more sunlight and water, making it healthier. Taller grass also keeps sun and water from getting down to weeds, which helps keep undesirable plants at bay. Leaving grass clippings on the lawn after mowing naturally infuses beneficial nitrogen back into your soil.

3. **Consider a push reel lawn mower that's powered by you instead of one that uses gas, electricity or batteries.** This way, you'll avoid inhaling any fumes and save money too. These mowers are incredibly quiet—listen to the birds chirp while you mow! As an added bonus, your neighbors will be able to enjoy their backyard BBQ in peace. New lines of manual or reel push mowers are effective and easier to use than you might imagine, although sometimes the lawn needs to be mowed a little more frequently when you use these. Think of it as added exercise.

4. **Eliminate all-grass lawns and landscape with woodchips, rocks and native plants instead.** These diverse yards can be more beautiful than an all-grass lawn. They're also low maintenance and should do well without chemicals. Plus, this type of landscaping will help cut down your water bill.

5. **Plant native plants and rain gardens.** Native plants are easy to take care of because nature designed them to thrive in your particular climate and environmental conditions. Rain gardens consist of native plants and grasses with long roots. They're planted in areas where water might tend to flow or where there's a shallow dip. Rain gardens naturally capture and filter water runoff. Some local governments have resources—and even funding in some cases—to help you design and plant a rain garden that will thrive in your area. A local plant store or landscaping business might have ideas, and you can also find many instructions and tips online.

6. **Use natural compost or an organic, phosphate-free fertilizer.** Composting uses everyday materials—coffee grounds, eggshells, food leftovers, yard waste and more—that are gathered to decompose, often in a backyard. The result is a nutrient-rich material that can be spread on lawns and gardens and that naturally does wonders for plant life. Composting is easy, and many composting options and resources are available, including an EPA website: *www2.epa.gov/recycle/composting-home*. If composting isn't your thing, and you feel a fertilizer is necessary, go for one that's organic and phosphate free.

7. **Cultivate natural pest control.** As the saying goes, "The enemy of my enemy is my friend." So hang bird feeders, leave outdoor spiders alone and bring in or attract ladybugs (marigolds, cilantro and dill are a few plants ladybugs love) to control unwelcome bugs. Some plants deter certain pests. For instance, many bugs don't like the scent of marigolds, and basil keeps away mosquitoes, aphids and mites.

8. **Love your earthworms.** Avoid chemical treatments on your lawn so those helpful earthworms can thrive and naturally aerate your lawn without your doing a thing.

9. **Learn more about organic gardening**, which uses natural methods, and plant diversely to maintain a healthy lawn and garden. One helpful resource is *www.seedsofchange.com*. See the "Learning Center" tab for gardening tips.

10. **Buy garden hoses that are made from natural rubber or polyurethane and that are free of PVC and lead.** Before buying new garden products, do a little research. Kids often drink from hoses or run through sprinklers hooked up to hoses, and a study from HealthyStuff.org found high levels of lead, phthalates and BPA in hose water after the hoses sat in the sun for a few days.[110] The organization tested nearly 200 garden products (including hoses, garden gloves, kneeling pads and garden tools) for materials such as lead, cadmium, bromine, chlorine, phthalates and BPA. Researchers found 70 percent of the items contained enough chemicals of concern to be considered a "high concern," according to their ranking system. See *www.healthystuff.org* to find how various garden products rated.

GARAGE

. . . .

"Truth is by nature self-evident. As soon as you remove the cobwebs of ignorance that surround it, it shines clear."
—MAHATMA GANDHI

Garages are easy to ignore, but they warrant some thought and care. They're usually close to indoor living spaces, and the most potent chemicals and materials in a household are often stored in the garage. Fumes are easily sucked into homes through poor ventilation or as a back door is opened and closed.

1. **Evaluate and eliminate chemicals—and then stop buying them.** Many chemicals aren't really necessary, and a little research can often turn up a safer alternative for those products you truly need. Contact your city or county government or consult *www.earth911.com* to find a place to properly dispose of chemicals. Dumping them or tossing them in the trash does major damage to our water systems, soil and air, which ultimately harms human health.

2. **Store chemicals safely.** Keep them high up on a shelf so they're well out of reach of kids. Consult *earth911.com* for more details on proper storage.

3. **Back your car out of the garage as soon as you start it.**

4. **Consider a foil vapor barrier between your garage and house and make sure the seals around the door to your garage are solid.** This will help block pollutants from getting sucked into your house, including those that continue to release after a car engine is turned off.

5. **After a long drive, keep your car outside for a bit before bringing it into the garage.** Cars emit pollutants after they're turned off, so letting the car cool and sit outside keeps those chemicals from sitting in your garage and getting into your home.

6. **Add a yearly garage cleaning to your calendar.** Clean out the dust and cobwebs to keep allergens to a minimum. Consider testing drywall or susceptible areas of the garage for mold at this time.

CARS

• • • • • • •

"The winners in life treat their body as if it were a magnificent spacecraft that gives them the finest transportation and endurance for their lives."
—DENIS WAITLEY

That new-car smell is the scent of chemicals off-gassing inside a vehicle. Hundreds of chemicals are used in materials that make up the dashboard, steering wheel, seats, armrests and more. Cars and car seats emit these chemicals into the air you breathe. The problem of contaminated air is compounded inside vehicles because they're enclosed spaces. Also, more VOCs are usually emitted when materials are exposed to heat and sun, which cars often are. Fortunately, some cars and carseats are healthier than others.

1. **Use the HealthyStuff.org website to research the healthiest cars.** Download the organization's most recent car guide by searching at *www.healthystuff.org/departments/cars*. Researchers found more than 275 chemicals inside vehicles, including chemicals associated with birth defects, impaired learning, liver toxicity and cancer.

   According to the HealthyStuff.org car report, "Since 1960 the quantity of plastics used in vehicles has grown ten-fold, rising from 22 pounds in 1960 to over 250 pounds today. Many synthetic materials and plastics are produced with chemical additives that are used to change the engineering performance of the plastics, thus these plastics may contain plasticizers, stabilizers, flame retardants, antimicrobials and antioxidants. Due to these additives, many pollutants, including benzene, toluene and xylene, were found in levels exceeding indoor and outdoor air quality standards."[111]

The HealthyStuff.org report ranks vehicle companies, as well as specific makes and models. Honda has been the organization's top-ranked company—for being the healthiest choice for vehicles—since 2007.

2. **Search HealthyStuff.org for the healthiest car seats.** Researchers with HealthyStuff.org found that companies routinely make car seats using materials and chemicals that are linked to reproductive problems, developmental and learning disabilities, hormone imbalances and cancer. Babies and kids spend a lot of time in car seats, during which they breathe in off-gassing chemicals and touch unhealthy coatings.

A HealthyStuff.org study of more than 150 car seats from 2011 showed that 44 percent used brominated flame retardants that have been shown to be toxic or that lack adequate health-safety data. The study also found that 60 models contained one or more hazardous chemicals, including PVC, brominated flame retardants and heavy metals.[112] When some of these materials are exposed to sun and heat, they might emit even more VOCs into the air or break down into more harmful substances. Learn more by searching for the report on HealthyStuff.org or see the best and worst models from 2011 at *www.healthystuff.org/bw.080311.carseats.php*

COUNTERTOPS

* * * * * * *

*"You learn a lot about someone
when you share a meal together."*
—ANTHONY BOURDAIN

When you're remodeling or building a home, avoid the pitfalls of many countertop materials, which commonly use plastics, off-gas VOCs, contain glues with formaldehyde or require routine chemical coatings, sealants and maintenance products.

1. **When remodeling or building, look for natural materials and research the resins and coatings as well.** Some good options use recycled glass, recycled paper, bamboo and even walnut shells. Make sure all the materials, including glues, resins, sealants and coatings, are free of VOCs and formaldehyde. Look for something that states it does not off-gas.

2. **Be aware that granite and other stone-based countertops may emit low levels of radon and radiation.** Although the EPA says the levels that are likely released from countertops are probably lower than what's emitted from other sources,[113] it's still something worth considering.

CONSTRUCTION, HOME BUILDING AND REMODELING

. . . .

"Peace is a daily, a weekly, a monthly process, gradually changing opinions, slowly eroding old barriers, quietly building new structures."
—JOHN F. KENNEDY

Whether you're doing small projects around the house, building a home from the ground up or remodeling a room or two, keep these tips and resources in mind.

1. **The rule of thumb is that natural materials are generally healthier.** Wherever you can choose items that are closer to nature, do so.

2. **Keep construction projects separate from family living.** Even minor construction should take place while children, and anyone else who isn't necessary for the project, are out of the home. This minimizes people's exposure to materials that off-gas and to miniscule building materials that end up floating in the air.

3. **Keep projects tidy.** Close off rooms that aren't undergoing construction and open windows to ventilate the rooms where projects are taking place. Even if you're working on something small, it's important to take precautions.

4. **Clean up thoroughly.** You might not be able to see or smell the effects of a project, but it's important to include careful cleaning as a last step. Use a vacuum with a HEPA filter to clean the entire surrounding area, and then dust and mop with a wet cloth.

5. **Check out these resources for healthier building and remodeling:**
   - Environmental Protection Agency's Energy Star program, for greener, more efficient homes:
   www.energystar.gov
   - Environmental Protection Agency's Indoor airPLUS program:
   www.epa.gov/iaplus01/
   - GreenDepot, which has green building supply showrooms across the country:
   www.greendepot.com
   - The Healthy House Institute, for consumer information on making homes healthier:
   www.healthyhouseinstitute.com
   - U.S. Green Building Council's Green Home Guide, connecting consumers to ideas, advice and green home professionals:
   www.greenhomeguide.com
   - U.S. Green Building Council's LEED certification, an internationally recognized green building program:
   www.new.usgbc.org/leed

6. **Find a local business that specializes in healthier home remodeling, and purchase your materials from them.** Here are some examples:
   - Amicus Green Building Center, Kensington, Maryland
   www.amicusgreen.com
   - Build It Naturally, Asheville, North Carolina
   www.builditnaturally.com
   - Common Ground, Durham, North Carolina
   www.commongroundgreen.com
   - Dwell Smart, Charleston, South Carolina
   www.dwellsmart.com
   - Eco Simplista, Fort Lauderdale, Florida
   www.ecosimplista.com

- Green Space, Santa Cruz, California
  www.greenspacecompany.com
- Green Works Building Supply, Vancouver, British Columbia, Canada
  www.greenworksbuildingsupply.com
- The Healthiest Home, Ottawa, Ontario, Canada
  www.thehealthiesthome.com
- House & Earth, Austin, Texas
  www.houseandearth.com
- Natural Built Home, Minneapolis, Minnesota
  www.naturalbuilthome.com
- Nature Neutral, Charlottesville, Virginia
  www.natureneutral.com
- Tree House, Austin, Texas
  www.treehouseonline.com

ELECTROMAGNETIC FIELDS (EMF)

• • • • • • •

"The goal of life is to make your heartbeat match the beat of the universe, to match your nature with Nature."
—JOSEPH CAMPBELL

The idea that people have invisible energy fields and that the balance of our energy plays an important role in health is ages old—it's what terms like chi, prana, shakti and chakras refer to and it's what healing modalities like acupuncture, yoga, Qigong and Reiki address. What people knew intuitively thousands of years ago—that we're all energetic beings, and that disrupted energy can cause poor health—science is now showing.

Modern technology allows us to see some of the energetic, or electrical, vibrations and waves throughout the body. For instance, the electroencephalogram (EEG) shows the electrical communication among neurons in the brain (brain waves). The electrocardiogram (EKG and ECG) shows the electrical system that powers a heartbeat. This natural energetic or electrical force isn't unique to the brain and heart. Rather, each cell in your body has an electrical force that helps regulate complex biochemical interactions and processes that keep your body running properly.

As energetic beings, people also naturally produce subtle electromagnetic fields. These naturally occurring EMFs are miniscule compared with the EMFs created by recent man-made technology, including cellphones, WiFi, power lines, TVs and appliances.

Concern is growing about the sudden onslaught of strong EMF

exposure in recent decades—these new, powerful waves may disrupt humans' subtle vibrations and electromagnetic systems. One example is a cellphone, which is like a strong radio that sends signals (waves) to a faraway station. Those waves can also penetrate brain tissue, organs and other parts of your body.

EMFs have the potential to interfere with how cells in your body communicate with one another, inhibit your cells ability to detoxify and repair themselves, create a stress response in the body and affect hormone levels.

Even when wireless devices like cellphones aren't in use, they're constantly touching base with a far-off signal when they're on, so they're still giving off EMFs. Other electrical devices, such as appliances, can continuously emit some EMFs if they're plugged in.

Some health experts who study EMFs refer to them as a risky experiment on humankind. And some experts estimate that people today are exposed to 100 million times more EMFs than their grandparents. It may be many more decades before there's more clarity around the consequences of that. And in the meantime, it's easy to be confused about this topic, as many studies are conflicting, and others are "inconclusive."

A smart consumer should be aware of some of the reasons it's been difficult to clearly demonstrate the health effects of EMF exposure:

- Everyone on Earth is constantly exposed to EMFs (because of satellites and other wide-reaching technologies), but some people are exposed more and others less based on their location and personal use of various technologies.
- Some of the health effects from EMFs can take decades to develop. Brain tumors, for instance, are often 20 to 30 years or more in the making. Studies usually span far shorter time frames and are therefore have a limited ability to capture longer-term consequences.
- Technology is constantly changing and advancing. That means a study involving cellphone technology from even a couple years ago might be outdated or fail to reflect current exposure levels.
- As each year goes by, more people use these technologies, people who have the technology use it more and younger children use more gadgets. This means exposure estimates quickly become out of date.

- Many studies on EMF exposure and health effects are funded by the technology industry. This presents a huge conflict of interest, as the industries and individuals benefit from the profit and convenience of new technology—and don't benefit when studies deem new technology unsafe.

Despite the many obstacles to research, consequences of EMF exposure have shown up:

- A study published in The Journal of the American Medical Association showed through brain scans that cellphone use changes brain activity nearest to the phone's antenna. Researchers concluded, "50-minute cell phone exposure was associated with increased brain glucose metabolism in the region closest to the antenna."[114] Although the exact consequences of this particular change aren't clear, the research proves that cellphones affect brain activity.
- In 2011, the World Health Organization and its International Agency for Research on Cancer (IARC) classified radiofrequency electromagnetic fields, which are present in cellphones (among other technologies), as "possibly carcinogenic to humans" due to the increased risk for glioma, a malignant form of brain cancer, which is associated with wireless phone use.[115]
- More than one meta-analysis of studies shows an association between cellphone use and an increased risk for certain types of brain cancer: glioma and acoustic neuroma.[116] One of the studies concludes, "Our analysis of the literature studies and of the results from meta-analyses of the significant data alone shows an almost doubling of the risk of head tumours induced by long-term mobile phone use or latency."[117]
- The IARC's international Interphone study found that the risk for brain tumors was higher in people who used cellphones most—at least 30 minutes a day—and in people who had been using them for the longest period of time—at least 10 years.[118]
- A study of early adolescents' use of cell phones concluded that, "If their use continued at the reported rate, many would be at increased risk of specific brain tumours by their mid-teens [...]."[119]
- Multiple studies indicate that cellphone radiation damages

human sperm.[120] [121] One review of the studies concluded that exposure decreases sperm concentration, quality and viability. "These abnormalities seem to be directly related to the duration of mobile phone use," researchers stated.[122]

- A study from UCLA's School of Public Health showed that "exposure to cell phones prenatally—and, to a lesser degree, postnatally—was associated with behavioral difficulties such as emotional and hyperactivity problems around the age of school entry."[123]

If you don't want to wait decades for crystal-clear evidence on EMFs' potential health consequences, you can take steps now to limit your exposure.

1. **Limit cellphone use and use a landline whenever possible.** Keep at least one corded landline in your house to use for longer conversations.

2. **When using a cellphone or a cordless phone, choose the speakerphone setting or talk with a wired headset.** This will help lower exposure to your brain.

3. **Keep your cellphone away from your ear, especially when placing a call.** The farther you keep it from your body, the better. Signals are strongest as your phone is dialing or ringing to reach someone, so at least hold it far from your ear until someone picks up. A careful read on your phone's manual will probably tell you the phone shouldn't be pressed directly against your body. Try to get into the habit of holding it an inch or more away from your ear while talking.

4. **Don't talk on your cellphone in the car or in places where signals are weak.** Talking in a moving vehicle gives you stronger exposure as your phone is constantly working to connect to the nearest antenna. If signals are weak, the phone is also working harder to connect, giving you more EMF exposure. In addition, talking on the phone while driving is distracting and puts you and everyone else on the road at risk. In light of the research showing that

talking on the phone while driving is hazardous, more states are outlawing the practice.[124]

5. **Turn your phone off or switch it to airplane/flight mode when you're not using it or while you're sleeping.** Find the airplane mode in your settings. This turns off the wireless transmitter so you can't make or receive calls or texts, but it still allows you to use the phone for other purposes, including as an alarm clock.

6. **Switch the side of your head on which you hold your phone.** This will reduce concentrated exposure to one side of your brain.

7. **Keep your phone out of your pocket (and anywhere else near your body) whenever possible.** The farther the phone is from your body, the better. If you have it on while at work, for instance, set it at the far corner of your desk.

8. **If you are pregnant, limit your use of cellphones (and cordless phones) as much as possible** and keep them far from your midsection when you do use them.

9. **Don't let kids have or play with cellphones, tablets or other gadgets that use wireless connections without first disabling all wireless connections.** Children's developing bodies and brains, and thinner skulls, are more susceptible to damage from EMFs. Their brains also absorb more radiation than adults' brains. And children also have more years ahead of them to suffer the consequences of accumulated EMF exposures. If you're going to let a child look at pictures or play games on a cellphone, tablet or other device, it's really important to switch it over to airplane mode (which can be found in settings) and turn off any wireless connections.

10. **Whenever possible, use a wired connection for Internet instead of wireless, and turn off your wireless when you're not using it (at least overnight).** If wireless is your only option, unplug the main device every night so you at least limit exposure while you sleep. The next day when you need Internet,

simply plug your wireless back in and hit the reset button on your Internet. Also, keep the equipment out of bedrooms or other commonly used rooms.

11. **Whenever possible, choose wired technology over wireless for printers, keyboards, baby monitors and other devices.**

12. **If you have a wireless baby monitor, keep it several feet away from your baby's crib.**

13. **Use a baby monitor with a voice activation setting.** This will also help reduce your baby's exposure to EMFs.

14. **Keep your laptop off your lap.** When it sits directly on your body, you're absorbing more EMFs, so at least set it up on a table or couch or away from you on the floor.

15. **Turn off or disable any wireless-connectivity software on your computer when you don't need the connection.** Otherwise, your computer may be constantly checking in with nearby devices.

16. **Keep babies, kids and yourself away from the microwave.** Stand away from the microwave as it zaps your food. Microwaves use the same type of radiation as cellphones.

17. **Use a toaster oven instead of a microwave.**

18. **Stay several feet from TVs and ensure babies and kids do too.** The farther you are from electronic devices, the lower your EMF exposure will be.

19. **When buying or renting a home, consider power line and cellphone tower locations.** The farther you live from these, the better.

20. **Keep your bedroom as free of electronics as possible** and use a battery-operated alarm clock instead of one that plugs into an outlet. Because you spend so much of your time asleep, it's especially important to clear out electronic devices from the bedroom.

Remove TVs, phones, electronic alarm clocks, heating pads and electric blankets. Some people find they sleep better with fewer electronics around.

21. **Look for appliances that say they're low on EMFs.** Some hairdryers, for instance, market this feature.

22. **Rent or buy a gaussmeter to measure how much EMFs various appliances and devices are emitting in your home.** This knowledge can help you rearrange items to reduce exposure. One place to find out more is: *www.microwavenews.com/emf1.html*

23. **Hire a building biologist** to evaluate the EMF exposure in your home and make suggestions for reducing that exposure.

24. **Visit the website *www.bioinitiative.org*** to learn more. The website includes summaries of research on EMFs and health.

RESOURCES

PRODUCTS

For healthier consumer products, including furniture, bedding, linens, kitchen supplies and more, try these websites:

www.coyuchi.com
www.eartheasy.com
www.greencupboards.com
www.greenhome.com
www.greennest.com
www.mossenvy.com
www.naturepedic.com
www.novanatural.com
www.ourgreenhouse.com
www.purerest.com
www.satarahome.com
www.soaringheart.com.

WEBSITES

Debra Lynn Dadd's website, Everything You Need to Know to Live Toxic Free
www.DebraLynnDadd.com

Debra Lynn Dadd's guide to the healthiest brands
www.debraslist.com

Earth911 website, for tips, resources, directions and news on recycling and other healthy home practices
www.earth911.org

EarthEasy: Solutions for Sustainable Living website, for green living guides, tips and products
eartheasy.com

Environmental Working Group's website, for information and tips on healthier home environments and products
www.ewg.org

Green Seal and GREENGUARD websites to find certified products, which are guaranteed to have met certain standards for health, safety and the environment
www.greenseal.org and www.greenguard.org

Green Living Ideas website, for healthy living tips
www.greenlivingideas.com

Green Science Policy Institute website, for up-to-date information about flame retardants in consumer products
www.greensciencepolicy.org

Healthy Child Healthy World website, for tips, issues and ways to get involved
www.healthychild.org

Healthy Home website, for healthy solutions for your home.
www.myhealthyhome.com

HealthyStuff.org website for background, tips and guides for reducing your exposure to toxic substances and choosing safer products
www.healthystuff.org

Microwave News website, for research and reports on non-ionizing radiation (one type of which is EMFs)
www.microwavenews.com

Scorecard, the pollution information site, to look up pollution issues in your town
www.scorecard.goodguide.com

BOOKS

Toxic Free: How to Protect Your Health and Home from the Chemicals that are Making You Sick, by Debra Lynn Dadd
www.amazon.com/Complete-Organic-Pregnancy-Deirdre-Dolan/dp/0060887451

Disconnect: The Truth About Cell Phone Radiation, What the Industry Is Doing to Hide It, and How to Protect Your Family, by Devra Davis
www.amazon.com/Disconnect-Radiation-Industry-Protect-Family/dp/0452297443

The Complete Organic Pregnancy, by Deirdre Dolan and Alexandra Zissu
www.amazon.com/Complete-Organic-Pregnancy-Deirdre-Dolan/dp/0060887451

Healthy Child Healthy World: Creating a Cleaner, Greener, Safer Home, by Christopher Gavigan
www.amazon.com/Healthy-Child-World-Creating-Cleaner/dp/0452290198

Beautiful No-Mow Yards: 50 Amazing Lawn Alternatives, by Evelyn J. Hadden
www.amazon.com/Beautiful-No-Mow-Yards-Amazing-Alternatives/dp/1604692383

Zapped: Why Your Cell Phone Shouldn't Be Your Alarm Clock and 1,268 Ways to Outsmart the Hazards of Electronic Pollution, by Ann Louise Gittleman
www.amazon.com/Zapped-Shouldnt-Outsmart-Electronic-Pollution/dp/0061864285

Super Natural Home: Improve your Health, Home and Planet—One Room at a Time, by Beth Greer
www.amazon.com/Super-Natural-Home-Improve-Planet-One/dp/1605299812

Green Housekeeping, by Ellen Sandbeck
www.amazon.com/Green-Housekeeping-Ellen-Sandbeck/dp/1416544550

Slug Bread and Beheaded Thistles: Amusing & Useful Techniques for Nontoxic Housekeeping and Gardening, by Ellen Sandbeck
www.amazon.com/Slug-Bread-Beheaded-Thistles-Housekeeping/dp/0767905423

The Naturally Clean Home: 150 Super-Easy Herbal Formulas for Green Cleaning, by Karyn Siegel-Maier.
www.amazon.com/The-Naturally-Clean-Home-Super-Easy/dp/1603420851

The Healthy Home: Simple Truths to Protect Your Family from Hidden Household Dangers, by Dave Wentz, Myron Wentz and Donna K. Wallace
www.amazon.com/The-Healthy-Home-Protect-Household/dp/B004WO9DNA

How to Grow Fresh Air: 50 House Plants that Purify Your Home or Office, by B.C. Wolverton
www.amazon.com/How-Grow-Fresh-Air-Plants/dp/0140262431

REFERENCES

1 An introduction to indoor air quality (IAQ), Volatile organic compounds (VOCs). Environmental Protection Agency.
http://www.epa.gov/iaq/voc.html

2 An introduction to indoor air quality (IAQ), Volatile organic compounds (VOCs). Environmental Protection Agency.
http://www.epa.gov/iaq/voc.html

3 Stapleton HM, et al. Serum PBDEs in a North Carolina toddler cohort: Associations with handwipes, household dust, and socioeconomic variables. Environmental Health Perspectives. 2012;120(7):1049.
http://www.ncbi.nlm.nih.gov/pmc/articles/PMC3404669/

4 The Safe Kids Buyer's Guide. Green Science Policy Institute. 2013.
http://greensciencepolicy.org

5 Biomonitoring Summary, Polybrominated diphenyl ethers and 2, 2', 4, 4', 5, 5'-hexabromobiphenyl (BB-153). Centers for Disease Control.
http://www.cdc.gov/biomonitoring/PBDEs_BiomonitoringSummary.html

6 Meironyté D, et al. Analysis of polybrominated diphenyl ethers in Swedish human milk. A time-related trend study, 1972-1997. Journal of Toxicology and Environmental Health. 1999;58(6):329.
http://www.ncbi.nlm.nih.gov/pubmed/10580757

7 Harley KG, et al. PBDE concentrations in women's serum and fecundability. Environmental Health Perspectives. 2010;118(5):699.
http://www.ncbi.nlm.nih.gov/pubmed/20103495

8 Chevrier J, et al. Polybrominated duphenyl ether (PBDE) flame retardants and thyroid hormone during pregnancy. Environmental Health Perspectives. 2010;118(10):1444.
http://www.ncbi.nlm.nih.gov/pubmed/20562054

9 Eskenazi B, et al. In utero and childhood polybrominated diphenyl ether (PBDE) exposures and neurodevelopment in the CHAMACOS study. Environmental Health Perspectives. 2013;121(2):257.
http://www.ncbi.nlm.nih.gov/pubmed/23154064

10 President's Cancer Panel. Reducing Environmental Cancer Risk, 2008-2009 Annual Report.
http://deainfo.nci.nih.gov/advisory/pcp/annualreports/pcp08-09rpt/PCP_Report_08-09_508.pdf

11 Lee DH, et al. A strong dose-response relation between serum concentrations of persistent organic pollutants and diabetes: results from the National Health and Examination Survey 1999-2002. Diabetes Care. 2006;29(7):1638.
http://www.ncbi.nlm.nih.gov/pubmed/16801591

12 Nash D, et al. Blood lead, blood pressure, and hypertension in perimenopausal and postmenopausal women. Journal of the American Medical Association. 2003;289(12):1523.
http://www.ncbi.nlm.nih.gov/pubmed/12672769

13 Abhyankar LN, et al. Arsenic exposure and hypertension: a systematic review. Environmental Health Perspectives. 2012;120(4):494.
http://www.ncbi.nlm.nih.gov/pubmed/22138666

14 Goncharov A, et al. Blood pressure in relation to concentrations of PCB congeners and chlorinated pesticides. Environmental Health Perspectives. 2011;119(3):319.
http://www.ncbi.nlm.nih.gov/pubmed/21362590

15 Teitelbaum SL, et al. Associations between phthalate metabolite urinary concentrations and body size measures in New York City children. Environmental Research. 2012;112:186.
http://www.sciencedirect.com/science/article/pii/S0013935111003112

16 Solving the problem of childhood obesity within a generation. White House Task Force on Childhood Obesity Report to the President. May 2010.
http://www.letsmove.gov/sites/letsmove.gov/files/TaskForce_on_Childhood_Obesity_May2010_FullReport.pdf

17 Hoffman K, et al. Exposure to polyfluoroalkyl chemicals and attention deficit/ hyperactivity disorder in U.S. children 12-15 years of age. Environmental Health Perspectives. 2010;118(12):1762.
http://www.ncbi.nlm.nih.gov/pubmed/20551004

18 Weinhold B. More chemicals show epigenetic effects across generations. Environmental Health Perspectives. 2012;120(6):a228.
http://www.ncbi.nlm.nih.gov/pmc/articles/PMC3385447/

19 Pollution in People: Cord Blood Contaminants in Minority Newborns. Environmental Working Group and Rachel's Network. 2009.
http://www.ewg.org/

20 Swan SH, et al. Decrease in anogenital distance among male infants with prenatal phthalate exposure. Environmental Health Perspectives. 2005;113(8):1056.
http://www.ncbi.nlm.nih.gov/pubmed/16079079

21 Vinson F, et al. Exposure to pesticides and risk of childhood cancer: a meta-analysis of recent epidemiological studies. Occupational and Environmental Medicine. 2011;68(9):694.
http://www.ncbi.nlm.nih.gov/pubmed/21606468

22 Fourth National Report on Human Exposure to Environmental Chemicals. Centers for Disease Control. 2009.
http://www.cdc.gov/ExposureReport/pdf/FourthReport.pdf

23 Relyea RA. A cocktail of contaminants: how mixtures of pesticides at low concentrations affect aquatic communities. Oecologia. 2009;159(2):363.
http://www.ncbi.nlm.nih.gov/pubmed/19002502

24 Vandenberg LN, et al. Hormones and endocrine-disrupting chemicals: low-dose effects and nonmonotonic dose responses. Endocrine Reviews. 2012;33(3):378.
http://www.ncbi.nlm.nih.gov/pubmed/22419778

25 Birnbaum LS. Environmental chemicals: Evaluating low-dose effects. Environmental Health Perspectives. 2012;120(4):a143.
http://www.ncbi.nlm.nih.gov/pmc/articles/PMC3339483/

26 World Health Organization (WHO)/International Agency for Research on Cancer (IARC). IARC classifies radiofrequency electromagnetic fields as possibly carcinogenic to humans. May 31, 2011.
http://w2.iarc.fr/en/media-centre/pr/2011/index.php

27 Hardell L, et al. Use of mobile phones and cordless phones is associated with increased risk for glioma and acoustic neuroma. Pathophysiology. 2013;20(2):85.
http://www.ncbi.nlm.nih.gov/pubmed/23261330

28 Levis AG, et al. Mobile phones and head tumours. The discrepancies in cause-effect relationships in the epidemiological studies – how do they arise? Environmental Health. 2011;10:59.
http://www.ncbi.nlm.nih.gov/pubmed/21679472

29 Cardis E, et al, with the INTERPHONE study group. Brain tumour risk in relation to mobile telephone use: Results of the INTERPHONE international case-control study. International Journal of Epidemiology. 2010;39(3):675.
http://ije.oxfordjournals.org/content/39/3/675.abstract

30 Agarwal A, et al. Effect of cell phone usage on semen analysis in men attending infertility clinic: an observational study. Fertility and Sterility. 2008;89(1):124.
http://www.ncbi.nlm.nih.gov/pubmed/17482179

31 Makker K, et al. Cell phones: modern man's nemesis? Reproductive BioMedicine Online. 2009;18(1):148.
http://www.ncbi.nlm.nih.gov/pubmed/19146782

32 LaVignera S, et al. Effects of the exposure to mobile phones on male reproduction: a review of the literature. Journal of Andrology. 2012;33(3):350.
http://www.ncbi.nlm.nih.gov/pubmed/21799142

33 Divan HA, et al. Prenatal and postnatal exposure to cell phone use and behavioral problems in children. Epidemiology. 2008;19(4):523.
http://www.ncbi.nlm.nih.gov/pubmed/18467962

34 Khurana VG, et al. Cell phones and brain tumors: a review including the long-term epidemiologic data. Surgical Neurology. 2009;72(3):205.
http://www.ncbi.nlm.nih.gov/pubmed/19328536

35 An introduction to indoor air quality (IAQ), Volatile organic compounds (VOCs). Environmental Protection Agency.
http://www.epa.gov/iaq/voc.html

36 Antimony compounds. Environmental Protection Agency.
http://www.epa.gov/ttnatw01/hlthef/antimony.html

37 In the Dust, Toxic Flame Retardants in American Homes. Environmental Working Group. May 2004.
http://www.ewg.org/research/pbdes-fire-retardants-dust

38 Perfluorinated Chemicals (PFCs). National Institute of Environmental Health Sciences.
http://www.niehs.nih.gov/health/materials

39 Basis for educational recommendations on reducing childhood lead exposure. Environmental Protection Agency. June 2000.
http://www2.epa.gov/sites/production/files/documents/reduc_pb.pdf

40 Formaldehyde. Environmental Protection Agency.
http://www.epa.gov/ttnatw01/hlthef/formalde.html

41 Johnson PI, et al. Associations between brominated flame retardants in house dust and hormone levels in men. Science of the Total Environment. 2013;445-446:177.
http://www.ncbi.nlm.nih.gov/pubmed/23333513

42 Harley KG, et al. PBDE concentrations in women's serum and fecundability. Environmental Health Perspectives. 2010;118(5):699.
http://www.ncbi.nlm.nih.gov/pubmed/20103495

43 Chevrier J, et al. Polybrominated duphenyl ether (PBDE) flame retardants and thyroid hormone during pregnancy. Environmental Health Perspectives. 2010;118(10):1444.
http://www.ncbi.nlm.nih.gov/pubmed/20562054

44 Eskenazi B, et al. In utero and childhood polybrominated diphenyl ether (PBDE) exposures and neurodevelopment in the CHAMACOS study. Environmental Health Perspectives. 2013;121(2):257.
http://www.ncbi.nlm.nih.gov/pmc/articles/PMC3569691/

45 From Field to Store: Your T-Shirt's Life Story. Natural Resources Defense Council.
http://www.nrdc.org/living/stuff/t-shirt-life-story.asp

46 The Deadly Chemicals in Cotton. Environmental Justice Foundation in collaboration with Pesticide Action Network UK. 2007.
http://ejfoundation.org/cotton/the-deadly-chemicals-in-cotton

47 Triclosan: What consumers should know. Food and Drug Administration.
www.fda.gov/forconsumers/consumerupdates/ucm205999.htm

48 Pesticides in soap, toothpaste and breast milk – Is it kid-safe? Environmental Working Group. July 2008.
http://www.ewg.org/research/pesticide-soap-toothpaste-and-breast-milk-it-kid-safe

49 Council on Scientific Affairs, American Medical Association. Use of antimicrobial agents in consumer products. Archives of Dermatology. 2002;138(8):1082.
http://www.ncbi.nlm.nih.gov/pubmed/12164747

50 Aiello AE, et al. Consumer antibacterial soaps: effective or just risky? Clinical Infectious Diseases. 2007. 1;45: Suppl 2:S137.
http://www.ncbi.nlm.nih.gov/pubmed/17683018

51 Calafat AM, et al. Urinary concentrations of triclosan in the U.S. population: 2003-2004. Environmental Health Perspectives. 2008;116(3):303.
http://www.ncbi.nlm.nih.gov/pubmed/18335095

52 Blount BC, et al. Levels of seven urinary phthalate metabolites in a human reference population. Environmental Health Perspectives. 2000;108(10):979.
www.ncbi.nlm.nih.gov/pubmed/11049818

53 Swan SH, et al. Decrease in anogenital distance among male infants with prenatal phthalate exposure. Environmental Health Perspectives. 2005;113(8):1056.
www.ncbi.nlm.nih.gov/pubmed/16079079

54 Jurewicz J, et al. Exposure to phthalates: reproductive outcome and children health. A review of the epidemiological studies. International Journal of Occupational Medicine and Environmental Health. 2011;24(2):115.
www.ncbi.nlm.nih.gov/pubmed/21594692

55 Engel SM, etal. Prenatal phthalate exposure is associated with childhood behavior and executive functioning. Environmental Health Perspectives. 2010;118(4):565.
www.ncbi.nlm.nih.gov/pubmed/20106747

56 Duty SM, et al. The relationship between environmental exposures to phthalates and DNA damage in human sperm using the neutral comet assay. Environmental Health Perspectives. 2003;111(9)1164.
www.ncbi.nlm.nih.gov/pmc/articles/PMC1241569/

57 Teitelbaum SL, et al. Associations between phthalate metabolite urinary concentrations and body size measures in New York City children. Environmental Research. 2012;112:186.
http://www.sciencedirect.com/science/article/pii/S0013935111003112

58 Radon, Health risks. Environmental Protection Agency.
http://www.epa.gov/radon/healthrisks.html

59 An introduction to air quality (IAQ), Carbon monoxide. Environmental Protection Agency.
http://www.epa.gov/iaq/co.html

60 Guide to BPA. Environmental Working Group.
www.ewg.org/bpa

61 Swan SH, et al. Decrease in anogenital distance among male infants with prenatal phthalate exposure. Environmental Health Perspectives. 2005;113(8):1056.
http://www.ncbi.nlm.nih.gov/pubmed/16079079

62 Engel, SM, et al. Prenatal phthalate exposure is associated with childhood behavior and executive functioning. Environmental Health Perspectives. 2010;118(4):565.
http://www.ncbi.nlm.nih.gov/pubmed/20106747

63 Jurewicz J, et al. Exposure to phthalates: reproductive outcome and children health. A review of the epidemiological studies. International Journal of Occupational Medicine and Environmental Health. 2011;24(2):115.
http://www.ncbi.nlm.nih.gov/pubmed/21594692

64 Duty SM, et al. The relationship between environmental exposures to phthalates and DNA damage in human sperm using the neutral comet assay. Environmental Health Perspectives. 2003;111(9)1164.
http://www.ncbi.nlm.nih.gov/pmc/articles/PMC1241569/

65 Triclosan: What consumers should know. Food and Drug Administration.
www.fda.gov/forconsumers/consumerupdates/ucm205999.htm

66 Playing on Poisons. Harmful flame retardants in children's furniture. Center for Environmental Health. November 2013.
http://www.ceh.org/news-events/press-releases/content/playing-on-poisons-childrens-furniture-found-with-harmful-flame-retardant-chemicals/

67 Reducing your exposure to PBDEs in your home. Environmental Working Group.
http://www.ewg.org/pbdefree

68 Report on Carcinogens, Twelfth Edition, 2011. National Toxicology Program.
http://ntp.niehs.nih.gov/?objectid=03C9AF75-E1BF-FF40-DBA9EC0928DF8B15

69 The Mattress Matters: Toxic chemicals in crib mattresses. Clean and Healthy New York. November 2011.
http://www.cleanhealthyny.org/#!families/c1smv

70 Swan SH, et al. Decrease in anogenital distance among male infants with prenatal phthalate exposure. Environmental Health Perspectives. 2005;113(8):1056.
http://www.ncbi.nlm.nih.gov/pubmed/16079079

71 Jurewicz J, et al. Exposure to phthalates: reproductive outcome and children health. A review of the epidemiological studies. International Journal of Occupational Medicine and Environmental Health. 2011;24(2):115.
http://www.ncbi.nlm.nih.gov/pubmed/21594692

72 Duty SM, et al. The relationship between environmental exposures to phthalates and DNA damage in human sperm using the neutral comet assay. Environmental Health Perspectives. 2003;111(9)1164.
http://www.ncbi.nlm.nih.gov/pmc/articles/PMC1241569/

73 The Mattress Matters: Toxic chemicals in crib mattresses. Clean and Healthy New York. November 2011.
http://www.cleanhealthyny.org/#!families/c1smv

74 Volatile vinyl: The new shower curtain's chemical smell. Center for Health, Environment and Justice. June 2008.
http://chej.org/campaigns/pvc/resources/shower-curtain-report/

75 Poison in Paint, Toxins in Toys. Environmental Health Strategy Center. December 2011.
http://www.saferchemicals.org/poisonsandtoxics

76 Herdt-Losavio ML, et al. Maternal occupation and the risk of birth defects: an overview from the National Birth Defects Prevention Study. Occupational and Environmental Medicine. 2010;67(1):58.
http://oem.bmj.com/content/67/1/58.abstract

77 Environmental Working Group Cleaners Database Hall of Shame. Environmental Working Group. 2012.
http://www.ewg.org/cleaners/hallofshame/

78 Sherriff A, et al. Frequent use of chemical household products is associated with persistent wheezing in pre-school age children. Thorax. 2005;60(1):45.
http://www.ncbi.nlm.nih.gov/pmc/articles/PMC1747149/

79 Zock J, et al. The use of household cleaning sprays and adult asthma, an international longitudinal study. American Journal of Respiratory and Critical Care Medicine. 2007;176(8):735.
http://www.ncbi.nlm.nih.gov/pmc/articles/PMC2020829/

80 Swan SH, et al. Decrease in anogenital distance among male infants with prenatal phthalate exposure. Environmental Health Perspectives. 2005;113(8):1056.
http://www.ncbi.nlm.nih.gov/pubmed/16079079

81 Jurewicz J, et al. Exposure to phthalates: reproductive outcome and children health. A review of the epidemiological studies. International Journal of Occupational Medicine and Environmental Health. 2011;24(2):115.
http://www.ncbi.nlm.nih.gov/pubmed/21594692

82 Duty SM, et al. The relationship between environmental exposures to phthalates and DNA damage in human sperm using the neutral comet assay. Environmental Health Perspectives. 2003;111(9)1164.
http://www.ncbi.nlm.nih.gov/pmc/articles/PMC1241569/

83 Healthy Home Tips: Tip 9 – Use green cleaners and avoid pesticides. Environmental Working Group.
http://www.ewg.org/research/healthy-home-tips/tip-9-use-greener-cleaners-and-avoid-pesticides

84 Environmental Working Group to review formaldehyde releasers. Environmental Working Group.
http://www.ewg.org/guides/cleaners

85 An Introduction to Indoor Air Quality (IAQ) and Volatile Organic Compounds (VOCs). Environmental Protection Agency.
http://www.epa.gov/iaq/voc.html

86 Chemicals in Household Products. Breast Cancer Fund.
http://www.breastcancerfund.org/clear-science/chemicals-linked-to-breast-cancer/household-products/

87 Knight L, et al. Candles and incense as potential sources of indoor air pollution: Market analysis and literature review. Environmental Protection Agency. January 2001.

88 American Academy of Pediatrics Council on Environmental Health. Policy statement—chemical-management policy: prioritizing children's health. Pediatrics. 2011;127(5):983.
http://pediatrics.aappublications.org/content/early/2011/04/25/peds.2011-0523.abstract

89 Sathyanarayana S, et al. Baby care products: Possible sources of infant phthalate exposure. Pediatrics. 2008;121(2):e260.
http://www.ncbi.nlm.nih.gov/pubmed/18245401

90 Shea KM, American Academy of Pediatrics Committee on Environmental Health. Pediatric Exposure and Potential Toxicity of Phthalate Plasticizers. Pediatrics. 2003;111(6):1467.
http://www.ncbi.nlm.nih.gov/pubmed/12777573

91 Swan SH, et al. Decrease in anogenital distance among male infants with prenatal phthalate exposure. Environmental Health Perspectives. 2005;113(8):1056.
http://www.ncbi.nlm.nih.gov/pubmed/16079079

92 Jurewicz J, et al. Exposure to phthalates: reproductive outcome and children health. A review of the epidemiological studies. International Journal of Occupational Medicine and Environmental Health. 2011;24(2):115.
http://www.ncbi.nlm.nih.gov/pubmed/21594692

93 Duty SM, et al. The relationship between environmental exposures to phthalates and DNA damage in human sperm using the neutral comet assay. Environmental Health Perspectives. 2003;111(9)1164.
http://www.ncbi.nlm.nih.gov/pmc/articles/PMC1241569/

94 FAQs: Bans on phthalates in children's toys. U.S. Consumer Product Safety Commission.
http://www.cpsc.gov/info/toysafety/phthalatesfaq.html#ban

95 F.D.A. Makes It Official: BPA Can't Be Used in Baby Bottles and Cups. Sabrina Tavernise, The New York Times.
http://www.nytimes.com/2012/07/18/science/fda-bans-bpa-from-baby-bottles-and-sippy-cups.html?_r=0

96 Poison in Paint, Toxins in Toys. Environmental Health Strategy Center. December 2011.
http://www.saferchemicals.org/poisonsandtoxics

97 Vinyl chloride. Environmental Protection Agency.
http://www.epa.gov/ttnatw01/hlthef/vinylchl.html

98 Polyvinyl chloride (PVC). National Library of Medicine.
http://toxtown.nlm.nih.gov/text_version/chemicals.php?id=84

99 Stapleton HM, et al. Identification of flame retardants in polyurethane foam collected from baby products. Environmental Science and Technology. 2011;45(12):5323.
http://pubs.acs.org/doi/abs/10.1021/es2007462

100 One in Three Children's Toys Tested by www.HealthyToys.org Found to have Significant Levels of Toxic Chemicals Including Lead, Flame Retardants and Arsenic. The Ecology Center and Healthy Stuff.
http://www.healthystuff.org/release.120308.toys.php

101 One in Three Children's Toys Tested by www.HealthyToys.org Found to have Significant Levels of Toxic Chemicals Including Lead, Flame Retardants and Arsenic. Healthy Stuff.org.
http://www.healthystuff.org/release.120308.toys.php

102 One in Three Children's Toys Tested by www.HealthyToys.org Found to have Significant Levels of Toxic Chemicals Including Lead, Flame Retardants and Arsenic. Healthy Stuff.org.
http://www.healthystuff.org/release.120308.toys.php

103 Over Half of Low-Cost Jewelry Ranks HIGH for Toxic Chemicals Including Lead, Cadmium, Nickel and Chromium, New Study Finds. Healthy Stuff.org.
http://www.healthystuff.org/release.031312.jewelry.php

104 2011 Halloween Makeup Findings. Healthy Stuff.org.
http://www.healthystuff.org/findings.102611.halloween.php

105 Children's Sleepwear Regulations. U.S. Consumer Product Safety Commission.
http://www.cpsc.gov/PageFiles/98883/regsumsleepwear.pdf

106 An Introduction to Indoor Air Quality (IAQ), Pesticides. Environmental Protection Agency.
http://www.epa.gov/iaq/pesticid.html

107 An Introduction to Indoor Air Quality (IAQ), Pesticides. Environmental Protection Agency.
http://www.epa.gov/iaq/pesticid.html

108 What are Biopesticides? Environmental Protection Agency.
http://www.epa.gov/pesticides/biopesticides/whatarebiopesticides.htm

109 President's Cancer Panel. Reducing Environmental Cancer Risk, 2008-2009 Annual Report.
http://deainfo.nci.nih.gov/advisory/pcp/annualReports/pcp08-09rpt/PCP_Report_08-09_508.pdf

110 2012 Garden Products Study. HealthyStuff.org.
http://www.healthystuff.org/findings.050312.garden.php

111 2012 New Vehicle Study. HealthyStuff.org.
http://www.healthystuff.org/findings.021512.cars.php

112 2011 Childrens Car Seat Findings. HealthyStuff.org.
http://www.healthystuff.org/findings.080311.carseats.php

113 Granite countertops and radiation. Environmental Protection Agency.
http://www.epa.gov/radiation/tenorm/granite-countertops.html

114 Volkow ND, et al. Effects of cell phone radiofrequency signal exposure on brain glucose metabolism. Journal of the American Medical Association. 2011;305(8):808
http://jama.jamanetwork.com/article.aspx?articleid=645813

115 World Health Organization (WHO)/International Agency for Research on Cancer (IARC). IARC classifies radiofrequency electromagnetic fields as possibly carcinogenic to humans. May 31, 2011.
http://w2.iarc.fr/en/media-centre/pr/2011/index.php

116 Hardell L, et al. Use of mobile phones and cordless phones is associated with increased risk for glioma and acoustic neuroma. Pathophysiology 2012;20(2):85.
http://www.ncbi.nlm.nih.gov/pubmed/23261330

117 Levis AG, et al. Mobile phones and head tumours. The discrepancies in cause-effect relationships in the epidemiological studies – how do they arise? Environmental Health. 2011;10:59.
http://www.ncbi.nlm.nih.gov/pubmed/21679472

118 Cardis E, et al, with the INTERPHONE study group. Brain tumour risk in relation to mobile telephone use: Results of the INTERPHONE international case-control study. International Journal of Epidemiology. 2010;39(3):675.
http://ije.oxfordjournals.org/content/39/3/675.abstract

119 Redmayne M. New Zealand adolescents' cellphone and cordless phone user-habits: are they at increased risk of brain tumours already? A cross-sectional study. Environmental Health. 2013;12(1):5.
http://www.ncbi.nlm.nih.gov/pubmed/23302218

120 Agarwal A, et al. Effect of cell phone usage on semen analysis in men attending infertility clinic: an observational study. Fertility and Sterility. 2008;89(1):124
http://www.ncbi.nlm.nih.gov/pubmed/17482179

121 Makker K, et al. Cell phones: modern man's nemesis? Reproductive BioMedicine Online. 2009;18(1):148.
http://www.ncbi.nlm.nih.gov/pubmed/19146782

122 LaVignera S, et al. Effects of the exposure to mobile phones on male reproduction: a review of the literature. Journal of Andrology. 2012;33(3):350.
http://www.ncbi.nlm.nih.gov/pubmed/21799142

123 Divan HA, et al. Prenatal and postnatal exposure to cell phone use and behavioral problems in children. Epidemiology. 2008;19(4):523.
http://www.ncbi.nlm.nih.gov/pubmed/18467962

124 Cell phone and texting laws. Governors Highway Safety Association.
http://www.ghsa.org/html/stateinfo/laws/cellphone_laws.html

HOME ENVIRONMENT EXPERTS' BIOGRAPHIES

I am so grateful to the following individuals for their contributions to "Take Care: The Home Environment Guide." Biographies for all the experts who helped inform this series are on the website, *www.takecareguide.com.**

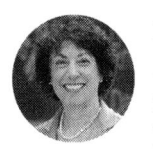

Linda Birnbaum, Ph.D., is director of the National Institute of Environmental Health Sciences, one of 27 research institutes and centers that make up the National Institutes of Health. She is a board-certified toxicologist and has served as a federal scientist for more than 30 years. She is the author of more than 700 peer-reviewed publications, book chapters, abstracts and reports. Birnbaum's own research focuses on the pharmacokinetic behavior of environmental chemicals; mechanisms of actions of toxicants, including endocrine disruption; and linking of real-world exposures to health effects.
www.niehs.nih.gov/about/od/director/index.cfm

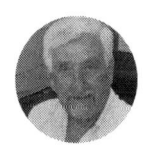

David O. Carpenter, M.D., is a public health physician working as director of the Institute for Health and the Environment at the University at Albany's School of Public Health. His research has focused on the study of human disease resulting from exposure to environmental contaminants. Carpenter, who received his medical degree from Harvard Medical School, has more than 350 peer-reviewed publications and has edited five books. Carpenter worked previously for the National Institute of Mental Health and the Armed Forces Radiobiology Research Institute.
www.albany.edu/news/experts/8212.php

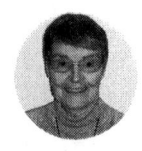

Theo Colborn, Ph.D., is an environmental health analyst and founder of TEDX (The Endocrine Disruption Exchange). TEDX is a nonprofit dedicated to compiling and disseminating scientific information on the health and environmental problems caused by low-dose exposures of chemicals that interfere with development and function, known as endocrine-disruptors. She is co-author of the book, "Our Stolen Future: Are We Threatening Our Fertility, Intelligence, and Survival?—A Scientific Detective Story," and has written numerous scientific publications on endocrine disruptors.
www.endocrinedisruption.com

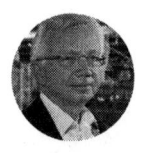

Richard J. Jackson, M.D., M.P.H., is a pediatrician and professor and chair of environmental health sciences at the Fielding School of Public Health at the University of California, Los Angeles. He has served as California's state health officer and director of the Centers for Disease Control and Prevention's National Center for Environmental Health. He co-wrote the books "Urban Sprawl and Public Health: Designing, Planning, and Building for Healthy Communities" and "Making Healthy Places: Designing and Building for Health, Well-being, and Sustainability" and hosted the 2012 TV series "Designing Healthy Communities."
www.designinghealthycommunities.org

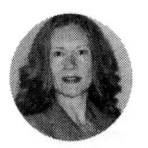

Kara Parker, M.D., is a faculty physician at Hennepin County Medical Center's Whittier Clinic in Minneapolis. There she co-created the Whittier Integrative Health Clinic, where she works as a primary care integrative physician. Parker is an assistant professor of family medicine and community health at the University of Minnesota, where she teaches integrative medicine to resident doctors. She is board certified in family medicine and holistic medicine and is on track for certification in functional medicine. Parker created and facilitates group visits to help people make lifestyle changes for optimal health. She practices healthy living with her family and uses her home as a "lab" for experiments in living well.
www.hcmc.org/providers/HCMC_STAFF_193

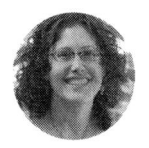

Stephani Waldron-Trapp, N.D., is a naturopathic doctor with more than a decade of experience in health care. She specializes in nutrition, weight loss, gastrointestinal health, women's health, children's health, fatigue, auto-immune conditions, detoxification, mental/emotional balancing and safe, effective pain relief. Waldron-Trapp owns and practices out of her private practice in Osseo, Minn.
www.naturalfamilydoc.com

*Please note that this book that covers many topics and points of view—the fact that these experts contributed information and insights isn't an indication that they all agree with every point in this book.

ALL CONTRIBUTORS IN THE TAKE CARE SERIES

Linda Birnbaum, Ph.D., is the director of the National Institute of Environmental Health Sciences of the National Institutes of Health and the director of the National Toxicology Program.
www.niehs.nih.gov/about/od/director/index.cfm

Dan Buettner is the founder and chief executive officer of Blue Zones, a company that uses evidence-based ways to help people live longer, be happier and become healthier by optimizing their lifestyle and surroundings.
www.bluezones.com

David O. Carpenter, M.D., is a public health physician working as director of the Institute for Health and the Environment at the University at Albany's School of Public Health.
www.albany.edu/news/experts/8212.php

Paul Chek, H.H.P., is founder of the C.H.E.K. Institute, which offers fitness and healthcare professionals a unique integrated and holistic approach to health, fitness and well-being.
www.chekinstitute.com

Theo Colborn, Ph.D., is an environmental health analyst and founder of TEDX (The Endocrine Disruption Exchange), a nonprofit dedicated to providing information about the health problems endocrine-disrupting chemicals cause.
www.endocrinedisruption.com

Marc David, M.A., is the founder of the Institute for the Psychology of Eating, a teaching organization dedicated to a forward-thinking, positive, holistic approach to nutritional psychology.
www.psychologyofeating.com

Larry Dossey, M.D., is a doctor of internal medicine, the executive editor of the peer-reviewed journal Explore: The Journal of Science and Healing and the author of 12 books on the role of consciousness and spirituality in health.
www.larrydosseymd.com

Henry Emmons, M.D., is a psychiatrist who integrates mind-body and natural therapies, mindfulness and Buddhist teachings, and compassion and insight into his clinical work and books.
www.partnersinresilience.com

Jill Grunewald, founder of Healthful Elements LLC, is a holistic nutrition and hormone coach with a focus on adrenal and thyroid imbalances and autoimmunity.
www.healthfulelements.com

Peter Hauri, Ph.D., was a psychologist and sleep expert who directed the Mayo Clinic Insomnia Program from 1988 until his retirement in 2000.
www.nytimes.com/2013/02/08/science/peter-hauri-psychologist-who-focused-on-insomnia-dies-at-79.html?_r=0

Mary Hayes Grieco is a spiritual teacher, speaker and author who directs the Minneapolis-based Midwest Institute for Forgiveness Training.
www.maryhayesgrieco.com

Mark L. Hoch, M.D., DABIHM, is the past president of the American Holistic Medical Association and a Bush Medical Fellow in Spiritual Healing based in Asheville, N.C., where he attends to the body, mind and spirit health needs of clients of all ages.
www.markhochmd.com

Richard J. Jackson, M.D., M.P.H., is a pediatrician, as well as professor and chair of environmental health sciences at the Fielding School of Public Health at the University of California, Los Angeles.
www.designinghealthycommunities.org

Elizabeth Lewis is a life coach, motivational speaker, certified stress-management teacher, licensed HeartMath Coach and approved teacher with the Midwest Institute for Forgiveness Training.
www.elewishealingarts.com

Stacy Malkan is an author and the co-founder of the Campaign for Safe Cosmetics, a national coalition of nonprofit groups working to eliminate harmful chemicals from personal care products.
www.safecosmetics.org

Bill Manahan, M.D., is assistant professor emeritus at the University of Minnesota's Academic Health Center's Department of Family Medicine and Community Health and past president of the American Holistic Medical Association.
www.holisticmedicine.org/content.asp?contentid=114

Jack McCann** is a sustainable farmer who founded and runs the Minneapolis-based cooperative True Cost Farm, which researches and implements the healthiest ways to raise meat and eggs.
www.truecostfarm.com

Rubin Naiman, Ph.D., is a psychologist, clinical assistant professor of medicine and dream specialist at the University of Arizona's Center for Integrative Medicine, as well as director of Circadian Health Associates, which offers sleep-related services, training and consultations.
www.DrNaiman.com

Janice Novak, M.S., is an author, speaker and wellness consultant who teaches posture workshops and seminars for hospitals, corporations and professional organizations.
www.improveyourposture.com

Kara Parker, M.D., is a faculty physician at Hennepin County Medical Center's Whittier Clinic in Minneapolis, where she co-created the Whittier Integrative Health Clinic.
www.hcmc.org/providers/HCMC_STAFF_193

Kim John Payne, M.Ed., is a counselor, an educator, an author and a researcher who directs the Simplicity Project, a multimedia social network that explores what connects and disconnects us to ourselves and to the world.
www.simplicityparenting.com

Greg Plotnikoff, M.D., M.T.S., FACP is an integrative medicine physician with advanced training in chaplaincy who practices at the Penny George Institute for Health and Healing in Minneapolis.
www.gregoryplotnikoff.com

Valori Treloar, M.D., C.N.S., is an author, a dermatologist, and a functional medicine practitioner whose clinic, Integrative Dermatology, is in Newton, Mass.
www.integrativedermatology.com

Carolyn Torkelson, M.D., M.S., is medical director of integrated health at the University of Minnesota Physicians Women's Health Specialists Clinic.
www.fm.umn.edu/faculty/torkelson/

Stephani Waldron-Trapp, N.D., is a naturopathic doctor who specializes in nutrition, weight loss, gastrointestinal health, women's health, children's health, fatigue, autoimmune conditions and mental/emotional balancing.
www.naturalfamilydoc.com

**Note: McCann is the author's brother

ACKNOWLEDGEMENTS

With deep gratitude, I thank my husband, Micah Moran, who designed the Take Care books and website and who has given heaps of time, energy, love and support for this project. *www.micahmoran.com*
Special thanks to Lisa Rummler, who skillfully and thoughtfully copyedited much of this book.
I'd like to acknowledge my dad, Mike McCann, for the author portrait and interior photos. *www.mccannphoto.com*
I really appreciate my fellow writers who offered their talents, suggestions and insights: Chandra Akkari, Phil Bolsta, Megan Ciampa, Mary Hayes Grieco, Jill Grunewald, Laurie Harper, Michael Kelberer, David LaVaque, Thomas Lee, Elizabeth Lewis, Lisa Rummler, Jeff Rush and Taylor Tagg.
Great thanks to my friends, family and acquaintances who provided feedback, ideas, resources and support: Maureen Araya, Bob Arnoldy, Mary Boom, Timothy Culbert, Anna Dvorak (*www.annadvorak.com*), Margot Fehrenbacher, Kate Foley, Alex Formuzis (*www.ewg.org*), Lori Fritzlar, Ann Garrity, Mary Kerns, Curt Kippenberger (*www.focusonhealthchiro.com*), Andrew Koss, Thomas McDaniel, Betsy McCann, Jack McCann, Jeff McCann (*www.mythicpaint.com*), Kathy McCann, Mike McCann, Phil Moran, Seth Moran, Susan Moran, Lynne Jensen Nelson (*www.naturalbuilthome.com*), Terry Pearson, Louis Slesin (*www.microwavenews.com*), Jennifer Simonson, Thomas Sult (3rdopinion.us), Mike Torvik, Molly Torvik, David Waletzko, Diana Waletzko and Colleen Ziebol.
Last, thank you to my children. You touch my heart, bring me joy and inspire me every day.

ABOUT THE AUTHOR

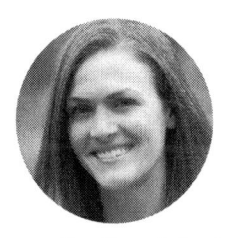

My health-writing career apparently started at age 4, when I posted lists of healthy foods on the family fridge. The pay wasn't so good. No matter—I'd realized a deep-seated belief that healthier is happier. I'd also discovered my interest in making it easier for people to make the most of life.

I've found the first step to any kind of growth is awareness. I believe one of the most powerful things we can do for ourselves is to notice what energizes us and what drains us. But in a fast-paced world full of confusing, conflicting messages about health and happiness, it can be hard to hear what our bodies and inner voices are trying to tell us.

Outside information and resources have often helped me get back to what I believe is already inside me—and inside everyone: the knowledge of what's truly beneficial. Distilling complex information into something useful became my professional focus. After graduating with a degree in journalism from the University of Missouri, I went on to write for newspapers, magazines and websites. My personal and professional interests intersected when I started writing about health and wellness for the Mayo Clinic, the Minneapolis Star Tribune, Experience Life magazine and others.

I started to notice the same themes continually running through health articles of all different types. So I decided to create a resource that connects the dots and reveals the basic, unifying principles of wellness. I wanted to make it clear why everyday choices matter and make it easy to take action. I hope the Take Care books and website, *www.takecareguide.com*, will do just that.

Thank you for reading.
Thank you for caring.
Spread the word.

―――

Wishing you true health and lasting joy,

Sarah

Made in the USA
Middletown, DE
20 July 2016